THE DOCTORS BOOK
OF
Home Remedies®
FOR
COLDS
and
FLU

Titles in
The Doctors Book of Home Remedies
series:

THE DOCTORS BOOK
OF
Home Remedies®
FOR
COLDS
and
FLU

Incredible Tips to Get You on Your Feet Fast— From *the* Leading Experts

By the Editors of *PREVENTION.*
Edited by Mary S. Kittel

RODALE

Cover Designer: Christina Gaugler

Library of Congress Cataloging-in-Publication Data

The doctors book of home remedies for colds and flu : incredible tips to get you on your feet fast—from the leading experts / by the editors of Prevention magazine ; edited by Mary S. Kittel.
     p.   cm.
  Includes index.
  ISBN 1–57954–210–7 paperback
  1. Cold (Disease)—Alternative treatment—Popular works.
2. Influenza—Alternative treatment—Popular works. I. Kittel, Mary S.
RF361.D63 2000
616.2'0506—dc21   99–055328

Distributed to the book trade by St. Martin's Press

2   4   6   8   10   9   7   5   3   1   paperback

Visit us on the Web at www.rodaleremedies.com, or call us toll-free at (800) 848-4735.

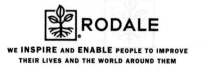

Notice

This book is intended as a reference volume only, not as a medical manual. The information given here is designed to help you make informed decisions about your health. It is not intended as a substitute for any treatment that may have been prescribed by your doctor. If you suspect that you have a medical problem, we urge you to seek competent medical help.

About *Prevention* Health Books

The editors of *Prevention* Health Books are dedicated to providing you with authoritative, trustworthy, and innovative advice for a healthy, active lifestyle. In all our books, our goal is to keep you thoroughly informed about the latest breakthroughs in natural healing, medical research, alternative health, herbs, nutrition, fitness, and weight loss. We cut through the confusion of today's conflicting health reports to deliver clear, concise, and definitive health information that you can trust. And we explain in practical terms what each new breakthrough means to you—so you can take immediate, practical steps to improve your health and well-being.

Every recommendation in *Prevention* Health Books is based upon interviews with highly qualified health authorities, including medical doctors and practitioners of alternative medicine. In addition, we consult with the *Prevention* Health Books Board of Advisors to ensure that all the health information is safe, practical, and up-to-date. *Prevention* Health Books are thoroughly fact-checked for accuracy, and we make every effort to verify recommendations, dosages, and cautions.

The advice in this book will help keep you well-informed about your personal choices in health care—to help you lead a happier, healthier, and longer life.

Acknowledgments

The following writers contributed to this book: Laura Catalano, Joanne M. Czarnecki, Staci Ann Sander, J. L. Sullivan

We would like to thank the following health care professionals:
Majid Ali, O.M.D., L.Ac.; Lee Berk, Dr.P.H.; Sheldon Blau, M.D.;
Rena Bloom, N.D.; Kenneth Bock, M.D.; Nancy Dunne Boggs, N.D.;
Bradley Bongiovanni, N.D.; Mary Bove, N.D.; Joan Clark; Franklin
R. Cockerill III, M.D.; Elizabeth Sander DiFiori, M.D.;
James Dillard, M.D., D.C., C.Ac.; Jennifer Dixon; Tiffany Field, Ph.D.;
Adriane Fugh-Berman, M.D.; Michael Reed Gach, Ph.D.;
Daniel Gagnon; Jay L. Glaser, M.D.; Richard T. Glass, D.D.S., Ph.D.;
Jane Guiltinan, N.D.; Elson M. Haas, M.D.; Willian Halcomb, D.O.;
Cheryl Hoard; Martha H. Howard, M.D.; Tori Hudson, N.D.;
Carol S. Johnston, Ph.D.; Feather Jones; Ellen Kamhi, R.N., Ph.D.;
Peter Katona, M.D.; Clifford Lowell, M.D., Ph.D.;
Allan Magaziner, D.O.; Ni Maishing, O.M.D., L.Ac.;
Gailen Marshall Jr., M.D., Ph.D.; Daniel B. Mowrey, Ph.D.;
Dean Ornish, M.D.; James W. Pennebaker, Ph.D.; Paul Petit, D.C.;
Joseph Pizzorno Jr., N.D.; Ronald L. Prior, Ph.D.;
Isadore Rosenfeld, M.D.; Wolfgang W. Shay, M.D.;
Katherine D. Sherif, M.D.; Adria Sherman, Ph.D.;
Andrea D. Sullivan, N.D., Ph.D.; Donald Sullivan, R.Ph., Ph.D.;
Varro E. Tyler, Ph.D., Sc.D.; Caroline Warner, C.M.T.;
Thomas G. Weidner, Ph.D.; Andrew Weil, M.D.;
David Winston; Susanne Wissell

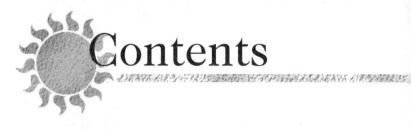

Contents

LETTING NATURE TAKE ITS COURSE 79

Annoying as they are, those sniffly, hacking, and achy symptoms are really your body trying to heal itself. Learn how and when to help it along in the fight.

STOPPING THE SPREAD 97

Whether a cold caught you or a flu bug bit hard, you *can* prevent it from attacking your family and coworkers, too—and keep it at bay the next time it comes calling.

ALTERNATIVE OPTIONS 111

Alternative healers are nothing to sneeze at. They offer a wide range of healing therapies that suit your specific cold and flu symptoms.

INDEX 121

Self-Care Is Key

It's Up to You

Got a cold or the flu? Well, don't blame yourself. It's not your fault that germs are everywhere.

Maybe you took a direct hit from the bank teller's sneeze. Or your toothbrush was too close to your roommate's germ-laced bristles. Perhaps at Saturday night's party you were drinking from a champagne glass that wasn't properly washed.

If you've caught a cold, it's but one of the estimated *one billion* colds "caught" each year in the United States. In fact, we don't really catch them. They virtually hurl themselves at us from every direction, as if we're a coach at tee-ball hitting practice. More than 200 viruses cause colds, which we contract easily by inhaling infectious particles placed in the air by other people's sneezes and coughs or by touching our eyes, noses, or mouths after touching an infected object or person.

When the influenza virus sweeps through a community, statistics show that 20 to 50 percent of the population are destined to become infected. Even if you're vaccinated each year, new strains of influenza are constantly forming. It's impossible to be protected from all of them. And if you get a shot, you can still pick up the flu bug within the 6- to 8-week window before the shot becomes effective.

You may have taken extra-good care of yourself this year, but getting sick was probably beyond your control. There's no need to suffer unnecessarily, however. With this book in hand, you'll discover how much ammunition is available to defeat a cold or flu. And chances are, you'll be able to do it all on your own, without having to go to the doctor.

Don't Wait for the Doctor

When it comes to taming a cold or flu, what can you really expect from your doctor? The truthful answer is: not a whole lot.

The National Institute of Health (NIH) reports that there is no prescription medical treatment available for the common cold, nor is there one on the horizon. Although many of the common rhinoviruses have been identified, it's not yet possible to identify or reproduce over 100 other cold viruses in a laboratory in order to create a cure.

Sure, you can find short-term relief in the hundreds of nonprescription cold products crowding the pharmacy shelves. But those syrups, pills, and sprays won't prevent, cure, or even shorten the duration of illness. Moreover, the NIH warns, "Most of these medications have some side effects, such as drowsiness, dizziness, insomnia, or upset stomach."

Medical treatment for the flu is nearly as nonexistent as cold treatment. The only drug doctors recommend for the flu is amantadine (Symmetrel) or its derivative, rimantidine (Flumadine). When conditions are right, it can reduce the length of the illness. Some doctors strongly encourage this drug for the elderly or people with impaired immunity—but they shouldn't depend on it. The drug is effective only for the Type A strain of the three major strains of flu, and to work it must be taken within the first 48 hours after onset of the illness.

Oftentimes, people in the early stage of a cold or flu make the mistake of asking their doctors for an antibiotic. While antibiotics make sense when a cold cascades into a "secondary" infection caused by bacteria, such as strep throat, they're ineffective for *viral* infections that cause colds and flu. So for the run-of-the-mill cold or flu, no antibiotic (no matter how strong) is going to help.

Antibiotics can also wreak long-term havoc on the digestive system, and when overused, they lower the body's natural ability to fight infections, warns Rena Bloom, N.D., a naturopathic physician in Denver.

The fact of the matter is, you're pretty much on your own. All you might end up doing by going to the doctor's office is swapping germs with other chronic coughers in the waiting room. But this doesn't mean that you should do nothing. At this very moment, you have a variety of proven, safe, and effective solutions at hand—the home remedies in this book, all provided by top medical and health care authorities. By making use of them, you have the power to suffer minimally—and cut the severity of your cold or flu in half.

Try This at Home

The best treatment for run-of-the-mill colds and flu is home treatment. Start by acknowledging that you're coming down with a virus. For self-care to work, you must respect your illness. Chances are, the longer you deny it, the longer it will take you to recover, and the more likely it will lead to a more serious illness such as a sinus, throat, or ear infection.

The first step of self-care for a cold or flu is to boost your overall natural defenses. Immune Enhancers on page 7 gives you 19 different measures to consider, from powerful herb and vitamin formulas to some unique stress-reduction techniques. You don't have to try them all; pick a few that appeal to you.

Next, get comfortable. Spoil yourself a bit. This is all part of the recovery process. As different symptoms develop, refer to Soothing Healers on page 31 for gentle solutions to feeling better—from old-fashioned chest rubs for relieving congestion to scented baths to take away chills and body aches.

Recipes and tips are in What to Eat and Drink on page 53, the center of the book, because what you nourish yourself with is at the core of your treatment. Conventional doctors and alternative healers alike believe that drinking plenty of liquids and eating warm soups are among the best things you can do to overcome colds and flu. We've picked the most effective, delicious, and soothing food remedies—from the kitchens of American family doctors to cultures that include India, China, and South America.

Part of the responsibility for taking care of yourself is having a basic understanding of your illness. Letting Nature Take Its Course on page 79 sheds light on *why* you're experiencing specific symptoms and how to banish them by listening to your body. As Bradley Bongiovanni, N.D., a naturopathic physician in Cambridge, Massachusetts, puts it: "Symptoms like fever, runny noses, diarrhea, sweating, and coughing up mucus are all functional and positive and are inherent to the healing mechanisms. Gently encourage your symptoms with natural therapies and common sense."

Sometimes we have no choice but to grab a decongestant or aspirin to get through the day, but in general, you'll recover better by letting nature take its course. In fact, often *enhancing* your runny nose or fever leads to quicker recovery and, ultimately, less suffering—because you're helping your illness move in the direction it's trying to go.

For example, a fever is your body's response to bacteria and viruses entering the bloodstream during a flu outbreak. When the body's temperature rises, disease-fighting white blood cells become more aggressive, and antibodies work faster. Therefore, suppressing a fever with aspirin makes it harder to eliminate the disease-causing organism and prolongs the sickness, says Dr. Bloom. Instead, this book shows you how to approach a fever by taking certain herbs that will "spike" it, then help it to come down naturally.

Better yet, this book even shows you how to outsmart a cold or flu bug by not getting sick in the first place. Stopping the Spread on page 97 offers a multitude of ingenious preventive measures. And there's an added plus—you'll also be helping to prevent those around you from getting sick, too.

When to Seek Help

There are occasions when home remedies don't work or aren't appropriate. The last thing you need is for pneumonia to develop from what started out as a simple cold. It's time to see a doctor when your symptoms last too long or when they are developing into a more serious illness.

It's time to call a doctor if you have these symptoms.

• Your cold is accompanied by a severe cough that produces green, yellow, or bloody phlegm.

• You have a sharp chest pain when coughing or wheezing.

• Shortness of breath, earache, acute headache, or facial pain develops.

• Your fever is accompanied by a stiff neck, severe headache, rash, confusion, back pain, excessive vomiting, excessive diarrhea, or painful urination.

• Your fever doesn't break in 2 days, or your fever surpasses 104°F.

• You have a chronic medical condition or are pregnant during a cold or flu outbreak.

All remedies in this book are prescribed for adults. Unless the tip states it, ask your doctor if the advice is appropriate for children. Most likely, dosages or measures will have to be altered.

Another reason to seek help is when you have reccurring colds or flu (such as more than four to six outbreaks a year). Perhaps this would be a good time to see one of the alternative practitioners listed in Alternative Options on page 111 who specialize in solutions that boost your overall immunity.

And remember that just because a treatment is "natural" or "herbal" doesn't guarantee that it's safe for you—in fact, some herbs can be toxic at the wrong dosage, and some have dangerous interactions with other herbs and drugs. If you're pregnant, don't use any herbal remedies (including aromatherapy) without consulting a doctor, because certain herbs cause undesirable effects such as early uterine contractions. You must also consult your doctor if you want to use herbal remedies but have a serious health condition, or if you're taking medications that could possibly interact with the herbs.

Although homeopathic remedies seldom have any side effects on their own, they constitute a unique approach that can bring about dramatic effects. If you use them in conjunction with other remedies such as aromatherapy, it's best to consult an expert.

Immune Enhancers

"The idea is to balance your immune system so that it's strong enough on its own to overcome the things to which it's vulnerable."

—Kenneth Bock, M.D., *clinical instructor in the department of family medicine at Albany Medical College; founder and director of the Rhinebeck Health Center and the Center for Progressive Medicine in Albany, New York; and coauthor of* The Road to Immunity

STAY WARM AND STAY WELL

*When your mother padded you top to
bottom in thermals and wool to keep you
from catching a cold, it really was worth
the scratchy-itchies.*

You probably learned one of the most important ways to
keep your immune system in good shape before you
were old enough to spell "influenza."

"Bundling up when you go outside in cold weather probably helps keep you from getting sick," says Clifford Lowell,
M.D., Ph.D. But even though being chilled might be a phys-
ical stressor, cold itself doesn't cause viral illnesses, he adds.
It's more likely that the wetness of a rainy or snowy day allows cold and flu viruses to get the better of you.

"We really don't have a perfect scientific explanation for
why keeping warm outside helps prevent colds and flu," Dr.
Lowell says, "but we know it's true."

So if you have to spend a lot of time in winter weather,
emulate skiers and lumberjacks. Start out with a layer of
long underwear made of a synthetic fabric that will wick
moisture away. Next, wear a wool sweater or fleece pullover
to create an insulation barrier. For your outer layer, consider
a coat made of water-resistant, breathable material like
Gore-Tex.

And don't forget Mom's last piece of advice as you were
leaving the house: Wear a hat. You can lose close to 50 percent of your body heat through your head.

—Clifford Lowell, M.D., Ph.D., *is the director of clinical
immunology at the University of California, San Francisco.*

EXERCISE COMMON SENSE

Staying in shape is a preventive measure to keep you from getting sick. And if you do get sick, working out can still be a good idea.

Regular, moderate exercise will enhance your immune system and decrease your risk of acquiring an upper-respiratory infection, says Thomas G. Weidner, Ph.D. But just because you already have a cold doesn't mean you have to turn into a couch potato.

If you want to work out while you're under the weather, the key is to reduce your intensity level, says Dr. Weidner, who studied 50 moderately fit students with colds. Those who ran, biked, or stairclimbed at 70 percent of their measured heart rates for 40 minutes got over their colds at the same pace as the nonexercisers.

On the other hand, if you work out to the point of exhaustion, your immune system could end up exhausted, too. According to a study at the Loma Linda University School of Public Health in California, more than 90 minutes of extremely strenuous exercise can make you more likely to become ill. Out of 2,000 people studied who finished the Los Angeles marathon, 13 percent came down with an infectious illness the following week. Of a control group who didn't run the marathon, only 2 percent got sick.

You should be particularly cautious about any exercise if you have flu symptoms such as fever, muscle aches, or a cough that brings up lots of mucus. In these cases, rest is best.

—Thomas G. Weidner, Ph.D., *is the director of the athletic training education program at Ball State University's Human Performance Laboratory in Muncie, Indiana.*

SLEEP IT OFF

Don't skimp if your body is pining for a pajama vacation. Otherwise, colds and flu might linger longer.

Deep healing takes place when you snooze. In fact, your virus-damaged cells recover mainly between midnight and early morning—this is because you aren't requiring your body to do much of anything besides heal.

"Getting plenty of rest is one of the things that most people know they should do, but often don't," says Clifford Lowell, M.D., Ph.D.

It turns out that your instincts to snooze are medically sound. At the University of California in San Diego, psychiatrists studied the effects of sleep on the immune system. They found that "natural killer" cells (immune cells that track down body cells infected by viruses and deliver lethal bursts of chemicals to destroy infections) dropped 30 percent in people who had just slightly less than their usual amounts of sleep in a single night.

An Australian study, showing the relationship between sleep and the immune response, found that vaccinated, but sleep-deprived mice were just as likely to get the flu as mice that were never immunized at all. The ones that had proper sleep, on the other hand, never contracted the virus.

In addition to getting plenty of shut-eye, taking some time off when you're getting sick rather than trying to work through it can really make a difference, Dr. Lowell says. "When we take it easy and take care of ourselves, we're much more likely to heal rapidly."

—Clifford Lowell, M.D., Ph.D., *is the director of clinical immunology at the University of California, San Francisco.*

DON'T LOSE SLEEP OVER SIDE EFFECTS

Read those labels. The pills you take to soothe yourself might deny you a night of healing sleep.

Over-the-counter cold remedies can help lessen your symptoms, but some can also make things worse in the long run. For instance, watch out for antihistamines containing pseudoephedrine, a chemical related to adrenaline that can make you jittery or keep you awake at night.

In any case, antihistamines might not even help you if you have a cold. "Colds are caused by a virus—not histamines, which are what cause allergy symptoms," says infectious disease specialist Peter Katona, M.D.

Also check to make sure your multisymptom remedy isn't full of caffeine, another product that can keep you from getting your Zzzs.

If you want your immunity to be at its best, prioritize sleep over pills, or use remedies with no side effects to relieve your discomfort.

—Peter Katona, M.D., *is an assistant professor of clinical medicine at the University of California, Los Angeles.*

DANCE IN THE SHEETS TO BOOST IMMUNITY

Having sex once or twice a week might strengthen your immune system enough to help ward off colds and flu.

An important disease-fighting component of the immune system, Immunoglobulin A (IgA), is the body's first line of defense against colds and flu. At any point in the body where bacteria or viruses try to enter, the IgA binds to the pathogens and signals the immune system to destroy them. It turns out that sex might boost this natural defense.

Psychologists at Wilkes University in Wilkes-Barre, Pennsylvania, measured the levels of IgA in the saliva of 111 students, then asked them about their sex lives. Those who had sex once or twice a week during the previous month showed a 30 percent increase in IgA over those who had been celibate. (Those who had sex *more* frequently than twice a week, however, had lower IgA levels—possibly because they were anxious about all the classes they were missing, and stress depresses immunity.)

According to Clifford Lowell, M.D., Ph.D., more research is needed to definitively say whether higher IgA levels will actually prevent you from catching a cold or the flu. . . but why wait? Just don't fool around once you actually *catch* a cold, of course, or you'll pass it to your partner.

—Clifford Lowell, M.D., Ph.D., *is the director of clinical immunology at the University of California, San Francisco.*

THINK ABOUT ZINC

Some consider zinc lozenges the wonder cure. Other people curse them. Many doctors say they're worth trying.

Zinc lozenges receive a lot of hype as a remedy that could possibly cut the duration of a cold in half. But why would you bother with this controversial mineral if some people report it delivering nothing but false promise—not to mention the reputation of having an unbearable flavor?

Let's put it this way: If you had a chance to suffer *half* as much coughing, headaches, hoarseness, nasal congestion, and throat soreness, would you suck on a little lozenge?

"Zinc helps support the immune system, especially since a lot of people are zinc-deficient," says Elson M. Haas, M.D., who takes zinc lozenges himself at the onset of a cold. "They work on a small or medium percentage of people who start taking them as soon as they get sore throats, and I've seen them work dramatically for a few people," he says.

Some studies have found that sucking on a zinc gluconate lozenge *greatly* cuts the duration of a cold. In a study at the Cleveland Clinic, 50 people who took zinc lozenges every 2 hours overcame cold symptoms 4 days sooner than people who took a placebo. In another study of 146 cold sufferers, people taking zinc recovered in an average of 3.9 days versus 10.8 days for the placebo group.

Then again, other studies have found no benefit to using the mineral. And some doctors warn that if you take too much, zinc might upset your stomach—not to mention your tastebuds.

Swallowing zinc in capsule form is no solution to zinc's unfriendly flavor, since capsules just won't have the same effect, says Dr. Haas. On the upside, rather than straight zinc, many companies offer zinc combined with enticing tastes like glycine or mint, or they even offer fruity-flavored zinc gum and lollipops.

But a word of advice—although they can mask zinc's medicinal taste, lozenges flavored with citrus or sweetened with sorbitol/mannitol seem to deactivate the mineral's effect.

—Elson M. Haas, M.D., *is the medical director of the Preventive Medical Center of Marin in San Rafael, California, and author of* Staying Healthy with Nutrition.

BE STEADY AT C

Recommending vitamin C to overcome common colds is as common among doctors as the common cold. But doctors say it's not enough to casually pop a few lozenges when you're sick.

How you take this famed nutrient really counts. Most important, make it a regular habit. When taken at the best time, in the best amount, and in the best form, vitamin C can best live up to its reputation as a tremendous cold fighter. Here are some guidelines offered by Andrew Weil, M.D.

• For starters, don't just start taking it when you feel sick. At the very least, a daily multivitamin with vitamin C will keep some in your system. Then if a virus begins to develop, vitamin C will be immediately available to help your white blood cells act more aggressively.

• The second thing to remember is that you should take it more than once a day. Vitamin C is a water-soluble vitamin, which means it leaves your body quickly. "I recommend taking it two to three times a day," says Dr. Weil.

• The amount to take has been a subject of controversy for decades. As a daily dose, Dr. Weil takes 250 milligrams two times a day. But when you're already sick, Dr. Weil is one of many doctors who recommend taking 500 to 1,000 milligrams *every hour or two* during the acute phases of your cold, and then returning to the 250 milligrams two times a day when you are well.

• Don't take more than your body can process. "You know you're overloading if you have flatulence or loose stools," says Dr. Weil. It's unpleasant, but nothing to be too troubled by if you reach that point, because the vitamin isn't toxic. Just cut back, making your regular dose just under the point that your bowels are bothered, he adds.

• Take vitamin C with food if you use it in pill form. Because some forms of vitamin C are highly acidic, they can upset your stomach, and some don't dissolve in the bloodstream. Better yet, Dr. Weil prefers the nonacidic powder form, calcium ascorbate. Stir it into a little juice or hot water and drink up.

—Andrew Weil, M.D., *is the director of the program in integrative medicine at the University of Arizona in Tuscon and author of numerous holistic healing books, including* Spontaneous Healing.

GIVE YOURSELF AN A

When you have a cold, vitamin A is a great benefit—so great that some doctors will advise increasing your regular intake by twentyfold.

You've probably been told to take the recommended daily value of vitamin A for your vision. Vitamin A is also a tremendous natural prescription for people coming down with a cold because it seems to strengthen immunity at the mucous membranes—staving off congestion, runny nose, and sore throat, says Elson M. Haas, M.D.

Dr. Haas recommends taking 25,000 to 50,000 international units (IU) of vitamin A three times a day for a few days when you feel a cold or flu coming on, then gradually cutting back to 10,000 IU three times a day for a few days when you start feeling better.

When you're not sick, stick to a daily dose of 5,000 IU. Unlike water-soluble vitamin C, vitamin A does accumulate in the body, so you have to be smart about how much you're taking—excessive amounts can cause toxicity. But you can take as much as 10,000 IU if you're particularly prone to catching a cold.

When you're ill, short-term use of extra vitamin A is fine, says Dr. Haas, provided you don't have a liver problem, aren't pregnant, and weigh at least 120 pounds. If you find yourself getting headaches or feeling a "band" around your head, cut back your dosage, he recommends.

—Elson M. Haas, M.D., *is the medical director of the Preventive Medical Center of Marin in San Rafael, California, and author of* Staying Healthy with Nutrition.

PUT MORE PRODUCE IN YOUR DIET

Loading up on fresh fruits and vegetables is an excellent choice of an immune-boosting program. It couldn't be much more simple or tasty.

Research proves that eating lots of produce keeps your immune system strong. According to a study by the U.S. Department of Agriculture—Beltsville Human Nutrition Center, a diet full of the powerful natural plant chemicals carotenoids raised immune-cell counts by 37 percent in 20 days. Carrots and squash as well as cooked tomato products are good sources of carotenoids.

It's also key to eat produce that can combat free radicals, which are dangerous chemical compounds that can harm the immune system. Antioxidants block the chemical reactions that generate free radicals and can help destroy previously formed ones.

United States Department of Agriculture (USDA) researchers at Tufts University in Boston found that the produce choices highest in antioxidant activity are prunes, blueberries, blackberries, kale, strawberries, and spinach. If you can't remember this list, going for fruits and vegetables with a variety of deep colors should provide ample antioxidants and carotenoids.

—Ronald L. Prior, Ph.D., *is the laboratory chief of the Phytochemical Research Laboratory at the USDA Human Research Center on Aging at Tufts University in Boston.*

TAKE A SHOT OF ELDERBERRY

Flu shots are good insurance. But if you forget to get vaccinated or pick up a virus anyway, elderberry syrup is a strong first line of defense.

Elderberry is a traditional European remedy used for hundreds of years to inhibit viral infection. Recent tests have scientifically proven this time-tested remedy. In studies at Israel's Hebrew University, elderberry syrup cut the duration of the subjects' flu in half, from 6 days to 3.

Elderberry provides a wall of protection around your healthy cells when flu germs come calling. It works by breaking down a certain enzyme that the germs would otherwise use to invade the cells and reproduce, says Andrew Weil, M.D.

You should be protected within 24 to 48 hours after ingestion, so take a shot of syrup as soon as you think you might be infected (flu symptoms appear within 2 to 4 days).

Products that say they are "standardized," taken according to the package instructions, so far show the best promise for cutting the flu short, says Dr. Weil.

—Andrew Weil, M.D., *is the director of the program in integrative medicine at the University of Arizona in Tuscon and author of numerous holistic healing books, including* Spontaneous Healing.

REPEL INFECTIONS WITH GARLIC

Garlic might chase people away from you, but it can chase colds away, too.

G arlic is incredibly helpful for the immune system in a number of ways, says Kenneth Bock, M.D., who recommends using it liberally as a general health booster. "Not only has garlic been found to have antiviral and antibacterial activity but it also enhances natural killer cell activity," he explains.

Natural killer cells are a mighty force in the immune system. They track down cells that are infected by viruses, then fire impeccably direct bursts of chemicals that destroy infectious microbes on contact.

According to Dr. Bock, you need to take large doses of garlic to have a medicinal effect. You can eat lots of it (see What to Eat and Drink on page 53 for remedies that use garlic in food), but taking capsules helps you monitor how much you get and is more pleasant if you don't like the taste in food. He recommends swallowing as many as 15 to 30 capsules per day for a few days when you start coming down with a cold or flu.

—Kenneth Bock, M.D., *is a clinical instructor in the department of family medicine at Albany Medical College; founder and director of the Rhinebeck Health Center and the Center for Progressive Medicine in Albany, New York; and coauthor of* The Road to Immunity.

DETOXIFY YOUR LIFE

You might not be ready to give up all your vices permanently, but taking a holiday from unhealthy habits can help strengthen your resistance to the viruses trying to get you down.

From a natural health standpoint, the most common reason for coming down with colds and flu is toxins, says Elson M. Haas, M.D. "Colds and flu represent the body's need to clear itself," he says.

When you're already sick, the last thing you need is a sausage sandwich with a soda and cigarette on the side. Your body has to work hard to rid itself of unhealthful substances. When you're trying to resist a bug, your body needs all its forces to heal, without siphoning off energy to move "heavy sludge" out of your system.

Having a cold is actually a perfect opportunity to give up smoking, excess sugar, caffeinated drinks, and processed foods—because you usually feel repulsed by these things when you're stuffed up and nauseated. Trust your instincts.

After all, caffeine-containing drinks are diruetics, which means that they cause you to lose fluid, worsening a mucus problem. An excess of sugar can lower the bacteria-killing effect of your white blood cells. Processed, fried foods are oozing with free radicals—chemical compounds that can damage the immune system when you need it the most. Cigarette smoke impairs your body's respiratory defenses against colds and flu viruses, and it also creates free radicals.

Giving up smoking and junk food for a while not only provides an easier opportunity for your body to restore itself but is also a positive step toward a more balanced lifestyle in the long run.

—Elson M. Haas, M.D., *is the medical director of the Preventive Medical Center of Marin in San Rafael, California, and author of* Staying Healthy with Nutrition.

TAKE YOUR COLD TO THE TROPICS

Hot, humid climates can do wonders for fighting cold infections. If you can't afford the ticket to Fuji, try a steam bath or sauna.

Spending time in a steam bath or sauna (preferably one with "wet" heat) is not only relaxing but also an effective way to help your body overcome a cold in a number of ways, says James Dillard, M.D., D.C., C.Ac.

"Although we don't understand the exact mechanism, we know that, generally, heat stimulates the immune system to help the body deal with infection—that's probably why we have fevers. Saunas and steam baths seem to assist in this natural defense," he says.

"In steam baths and saunas with steam, the steam dilates blood vessels in the infected areas. This encourages the white blood cells to get through the capillaries to the tissues, where they help destroy the virus," says Dr. Dillard. The extra humidity also contributes to getting you well, because it lubricates the mucosal tissues, allowing you to expel virus-filled mucus, he says.

You do need to follow a few precautions: Check with your doctor before taking a sauna or steam bath if you have health problems or are taking any serious medications. Don't go in if you've been using drugs or alcohol, because you could end up passing out. And be sure to drink plenty of fluids to replace what your body loses (as much as a quart of sweat per hour).

If you don't have access to a steam bath, a shower head such as the Misting Massage from Water Pik can turn your shower into the next best thing. Otherwise, just heat up a pot of water, sit with a towel over your head far enough away to keep from being burned by the steam, and breathe over the vapors.

—James Dillard, M.D., D.C., C.Ac., *is a clinical instructor at Columbia University College of Physicians and Surgeons and the director of alternative medicine for Oxford Health Plans in New York City.*

GET A MASSAGE

The right touch can raise more than your personal feel-good meter. It can also increase immunity. Massage is preventive medicine nobody minds taking.

Some people have the impression that massage only belongs in a hedonistic lifestyle, while others see it merely as a way to heal from injury. Sure, it feels great on a cruise and can help a bad back, but massage can actually boost your immune system, says developmental psychologist Tiffany Field, Ph.D.

It's not known how massage boosts immunity, but it could be because it lowers the body's production of stress hormones (stress hormones suppress immunity), or because the skin itself secretes an immune hormone that can be stimulated by touch.

Whatever the reason, it's a nice excuse to take a massage class with someone you'd like to get healthier with—or to ask for some tender loving care from a friend or partner.

Studies show that massage can boost immunity. But so far, no research shows it effective in reversing a cold or flu virus once it develops, so Dr. Field doesn't recommend it as a remedy for a full-blown cold or flu outbreak. Instead, make massage a regular part of your lifestyle and maybe you won't get sick.

—**Tiffany Field, Ph.D.,** *is a developmental psychologist and director of the Touch Research Institute at the University of Miami Medical School.*

TAKE A FRIENDLY COLD CURE

If you haven't been spending time with friends and family lately, you might be in for a rough cold season. Social connections help boost immunity.

It takes far more than eating right and getting enough exercise to be well. People who feel lonely or isolated are much more likely to get sick and stay sick than those who have a sense of connection and community, says Dean Ornish, M.D.

In fact, in a study by psychologists at Pittsburgh's Carnegie Mellon University, people who were married and had close friends and relatives were four times less susceptible to catching colds than people who had fewer social attachments. And the more diverse ties people had with friends, coworkers, family, and the community, the better they fared in fighting off a cold.

Dr. Ornish suggests having frequent meals with friends and family (that includes eating in the company cafeteria rather than camping in your office all the time). He also recommends making regular phone calls or even exchanging messages over the Internet to keep your social contacts strong.

If you are a stranger in a new community, consider volunteer work. Not only can it bring positive change to someone else's life but it also could keep you from suffering during this sniffle season.

    —Dean Ornish, M.D., *is a clinical professor of medicine at the University of California, San Francisco, School of Medicine; the founder and director of the Preventive Medicine Research Institute in Sausalito, California; and author of numerous health books, including* Love *and* Survival.

WATCH OUT FOR LONG-TERM STRESS

If you find yourself getting more colds, it might be all in your head. When negative thoughts and emotions make you tense, over time you weaken your immunity.

The common cold is one more reason to protect yourself against blood-pressure-raising, heart-harming stress. Chronic stressors such as unemployment or family difficulties substantially raise your risk of catching a cold, according to a study by Carnegie Mellon University psychologists in Pittsburgh. Fortunately, stressful life events lasting less than a month didn't make people more susceptible to colds. It's only the long-term tension that makes a difference.

Unfortunately, the researchers couldn't offer any findings on how to actually reduce this risk, apart from resolving the issues that are bothering you.

Fortunately, one psychologist offers a concrete solution that could help: Write your troubles down. James W. Pennebaker, Ph.D., asked students to write about either mundane topics or meaningful emotional issues for 15 minutes a day over 3 days. Those who expressed their emotions in writing increased the activity of their immune cells.

"In general, the more people are able to explore their emotions and thoughts, the better off they are," Dr. Pennebaker says. "While this doesn't necessarily mean you'll lower your chance of catching a cold or the flu, it's certainly worth trying."

—James W. Pennebaker, Ph.D., *is a professor of psychology at the University of Texas at Austin and author of* Opening Up.

LAUGH OFF
YOUR COUGH AND SNIFFLES

You know to lighten up because being stressed out can dampen your immunity. It's also true that a sense of humor can keep those virus-fighting cells in high gear.

It turns out that mirthful laughter produces "eustress," a *positive* stress state that helps reduce the immune-suppressing chemical reactions caused by everyday negative stresses, says pathology researcher Lee Berk, Dr.P.H.

Dr. Berk and his colleagues studied the influence of laughter on the immune systems of medical students at Loma Linda University School of Medicine in California. They found all kinds of benefits, including an increase in antibodies that help prevent infections in the upper-respiratory tract.

Their research used a video of the watermelon-smashing comedian Gallagher—which also seems to prove that future doctors enjoy seeing pieces of fruit fly more than most people. But you can get similar results from anything you actually find funny.

When you're sick, listen to Garrison Keillor, try on an outfit from the seventies, get sea monkeys—you know what tickles your funny bone. Do it. Even if your cold *doesn't* heal faster, chuckling will take your mind off your aches and pains.

—Lee Berk, Dr.P.H., *is an assistant research professor of pathology, assistant professor of preventive medicine, and associate director of the Center for Neuroimmunology at Loma Linda University School of Medicine in Loma Linda, California.*

SEEK SALUBRITY
THROUGH SERENITY

Rather than watching another rerun when you're home with a cold or flu, learning to meditate can improve your overall state of well-being and help speed your healing.

Meditation cuts down on your body's stress chemicals, strengthens the immune system, and helps you see things from a new perspective. "It's one of the most important things you can do to live a healthier life," says Dean Ornish, M.D.

While there are many religious doctrines that use meditation as part of their practices, the basics are quite simple and nondenominational.

- You can do it in any position, but it's usually recommended that you start in a seated position (chair or floor) that allows your back to be straight and is comfortable for at least 5 minutes.
- Now close your eyes. Repeat a soothing word (such as "silence" or "healing") in your mind every time you inhale, and as you exhale imagine your breath gently circulating through the parts of your body that ache or need healing.
- If you notice your mind wandering, gently bring yourself back to the meditation by focusing only on your breath. (If you're really distracted, try counting your breaths.)
- It's important not to judge yourself. All you have to do is be still, breathe, and try to stay focused on one image or idea, rather than succumbing to lots of random thoughts

that can lead to tension. It isn't easy, but you'll be amazed how healthy you feel afterward.

—**Dean Ornish, M.D.,** *is a clinical professor of medicine at the University of California, San Francisco, School of Medicine; the founder and director of the Preventive Medicine Research Institute in Sausalito, California; and author of numerous health books, including* Love and Survival.

AVOID ALLERGENS

When your allergies flare up, you're at greater risk for developing bad colds and, worse yet, secondary bacterial infections. Improve your indoor air and you'll reduce your risk.

You know that bringing lots of people together in sealed-up places can pass germs from person to person, putting a strain on your immune system. Making matters worse, closed areas in which ventilation is poor also lead to a buildup of dust and mold spores. These allergens, common in seasons when windows are shut, can lead to more problems than your normal sniffling and sneezing.

"Allergies make the mucosal linings moist and congested, which is a perfect breeding ground for viral and bacterial infections. Sinus infections and ear infections are particularly easier to contract when you have allergies because bacteria like the extra fluid filling your respiratory tract," says Kenneth Bock, M.D.

Underlying a lot of recurrent colds are allergy problems. And sadly, people are often given lots of antibiotics for sinus and ear infections. But if allergies are better managed, these other problems might be avoided, Dr. Bock adds.

The best thing you can do to overcome dust mites and mold is to use high-efficiency particulate arresting (HEPA) air purifiers. HEPA products were designed to remove 99.97 percent of all dust and mold spores, as well as pollen, animal hair, and dander.

Other tactics that might help are washing your bedding in hot water at least every 2 weeks. Consider using nonallergenic mattress and comforter covers and eliminating your feather pillows. Also keep up on your vacuuming with a machine designed to reduce airborne allergens.

Think twice about bringing firewood, which harbors mold, into the house. Instead, keep it outside until you're ready to use it. You can also help control mold by keeping your wet boots and shoes out of a closed closet.

Even houseplants grow mold in their soil, so remove them from your home if you're having problems. Of course, if you don't have a mold allergy, your favorite fern or ficus can also *boost* immunity. Plants not only put a tiny bit of fresh oxygen into the air but are also pleasant to be around, and they make people feel good. Keeping your spirits up can sometimes be as helpful to your immunity as keeping your windows open, Dr. Bock says.

—Kenneth Bock, M.D., *is a clinical instructor in the department of family medicine at Albany Medical College; founder and director of the Rhinebeck Health Center and the Center for Progressive Medicine in Albany, New York; and coauthor of* The Road to Immunity.

Soothing
Healers

"If you've caught a cold, your body is saying it needs a time-out. Let yourself have that, and do whatever it takes to make yourself comfortable and better."

—Andrew Weil, M.D., *director of the program in integrative medicine at the University of Arizona College of Medicine in Tucson and author of numerous holistic healing books, including* Spontaneous Healing

RELAX WITH MELISSA

Otherwise known as lemon balm, the herb melissa can lift your spirits not only with its bright, citrus flavor but also with its ability to ease aches. Combined with other herbs, melissa tea can rejuvenate you from the inside out.

According to seventeenth-century English herbalist Nicholas Culpeper, melissa "causes the mind and the heart to be merry." Melissa is an apt prescription for that all-around dull, achy feeling that sometimes arrives with a flu.

Herbalists have long recommended melissa for lifting foul moods, relieving tight muscles, and easing stomachaches as well as for its mild sedative effect. It also has antiviral properties that can fight infections associated with the flu.

Jane Guiltinan, N.D., prescribes a tea that combines melissa with Siberian ginseng, wild cherry bark, and echinacea. When combined, these herbs should put you in a relaxed, restful state while also boosting your natural defenses.

The echinacea blocks virus replication and stimulates the immune system. Siberian ginseng clears bronchial passages and reduces inflammation. Wild cherry bark and stevia are added for their pleasant flavors. Stevia is a potent natural sweetener, so if you find that the tea is too sweet, reduce the amount that you use.

Gentle Rejuvenation Tea

½ teaspoon dried melissa (lemon balm)
½ teaspoon Siberian ginseng root, finely sliced
½ teaspoon dried wild cherry bark
½ teaspoon dried echinacea leaves and stems
½ teaspoon dried stevia leaves
1 cup boiling water

Place the herbs in a tea ball. Steep them in the boiling water for 5 to 10 minutes. Drink the tea several times a day as needed.

—**Jane Guiltinan, N.D.,** *is a naturopathic physician specializing in women's health and immune system disorders. She is also a clinical professor and dean of clinical affairs at the Bastyr University Natural Health Clinic in Seattle.*

INDULGE YOUR FEET AND TREAT YOUR CHEST

Your feet are a long way from your tight chest and stuffy nose, but massaging them with decongesting essential oils is an effective treatment for your respiratory distress.

A romatherapist Joan Clark recommends massaging your feet with a combination of five essential oils—ravensara, eucalyptus, frankincense, pine, and cajeput. These immunity-boosting oils not only open up congested airways but also fight the infectious virus causing excess mucus. Frank-incense is especially effective at clearing up lingering chest colds, she says.

Just the act of rubbing your feet is recommended when you're sick, adds Clark. Aromatherapists say that a mere foot rub massages every major organ in your body, so it's a comforting treatment when you're grumpy with cold symptoms.

For the greatest benefit, use the specified portions and ingredients.

Breathe-Easy Foot Oil

    3 drops ravensara essential oil
    3 drops eucalyptus essential oil
    4 drops frankincense essential oil
    2 drops pine essential oil
    3 drops cajeput essential oil
    ⅛ cup carrier oil (jojoba, sweet almond, or apricot
       kernel)

In a small, dark container, combine the essential oils with the carrier oil. Cover the container and store in a cool place between uses.

Massage the oil mixture into your feet, taking extra time to work the oil into each toe and the balls of the feet (these are sinus and lung acupressure points). Wrap your feet in warm towels or heat them with a hair dryer set on warm to hot, which helps the oils penetrate more quickly.

Repeat this treatment as needed to relieve congestion. These are *medicinal* oils, so don't use them for more than 1 week without the guidance of a qualified practitioner.

—Joan Clark *is an aromatherapist and vice president of the Michael Schales School of Aromatic Studies in Los Angeles.*

SOOTHE A SORE THROAT WITH SANDALWOOD

When a scratchy throat turns painful, try a few drops of Mother Nature's aspirin.

The earthy and uplifting scent of sandalwood can bring a sense of serenity when you're feeling under the weather. That's not all. The essential oil of sandalwood can actually block pain signals to the brain, which is why it's recommended by aromatherapists as one of nature's aspirins.

Most essential oils should not be applied directly to the skin, but small doses of sandalwood are safe, says aromatherapy expert Cheryl Hoard. Just rub 3 drops of undiluted essential oil of sandalwood directly on your neck, wherever you feel pain. The aching should ease immediately, she says.

Although it will make you feel better, this natural aspirin won't actually fight the infection that is causing the pain. If you need antiseptic treatment, try the remedies in Letting Nature Take Its Course on page 79.

—Cheryl Hoard *is the president of the National Association of Holistic Aromatherapy in Boulder, Colorado.*

TAKE THYME TO BREATHE

*Sure, you know that echinacea and zinc
are popular for holding a cold at bay.
But once a full-fledged cold attacks, it's
thyme that is of the essence.*

If a cold virus progresses from the throat to the sinuses
(causing yellowish or greenish mucus), try the essential
oil of thyme, recommends aromatherapist Paul Petit, D.C.
This common herb is a powerful antiviral and antibacterial
agent. It is also good at clearing catarrh (inflammation) from
the respiratory tract and can relieve bronchial spasms.

Diffusing thyme oil in a potpourri pot or light bulb ring
carries tiny droplets into the air and deposits them where
cold and flu infection lurks—deep in the nose and the lungs.

Here is Dr. Petit's favorite thyme remedy, which includes oils of two other virus fighters—oregano and savory.

Thymely Decongestant

4   drops thyme (linalool) essential oil

3   drops oregano essential oil

3   drops summer savory essential oil

Fill a candle-style or electric potpourri pot with 1 inch
of water and add the essential oils. If you have only a light-
bulb ring diffuser, that's fine, but use just 1 or 2 drops of
each oil.

These oils are irritants, so do not ingest them or apply
them directly on the skin.

—Paul Petit, D.C., *is a phyto-aromatherapist and director
of technical services and clinical research at Phybiosis,
developers of natural health care supplies in Poway, California.*

BATHE THAT FEVER AWAY

You might not feel it while you're soaking, but essential oils of peppermint and lavender have natural chemicals that fight your virus. What you will be able to feel is blessed relief.

When you have a fever, holistic nurse Ellen Kamhi, R.N., Ph.D., recommends taking an essential oil bath over taking aspirin to bring down the body temperature quickly. "When the body increases its temperature, it is stimulating the immune system, keeping viruses from multiplying," she says. Allow the warm water to help your fever break in its natural way. The addition of essential oil can also help the process while making you more comfortable and stimulating your defenses.

Because peppermint and lavender are often used together by herbalists to reduce pain, they can relieve your achy-fever feelings. Peppermint oil also has a cooling effect that makes you feel relaxed while you wait for your fever to break.

Herbal Fever Bath

    3 drops peppermint essential oil
    7 drops lavender essential oil
    1 cup Epsom salts
    1 bowl cold water

Fill your tub with hot water—as hot as you can stand it. Then add the essential oils and Epsom salts. Place a washcloth and bowl of cold water outside the tub on the end where you plan to sit. Ease your body into the hot water and lean back in the tub. To cool your head, dip the washcloth in the bowl of cold water, wring it out, and place it on your forehead. Relax in the water for about 20 minutes. Re-dip the washcloth when you start to feel too hot.

When it's time to get out of the tub, make sure that someone is around to assist you. (You might feel lightheaded when you try to stand up.) Immediately wrap yourself in towels. Then climb into bed under lots of covers, and go to sleep.

—Ellen Kamhi, R.N., Ph.D., *is a professional member of the American Herbalists Guild, author of* The Natural Medicine Chest, *and host of several national radio and television programs.*

TAKE A CHINESE LOZENGE

Out of cough medicine? Sucking on gingerroot bathes the tissues of the throat with natural medicine to cure your cough.

The Chinese historically have used fresh gingerroot to ease inflammation and fight infection for a wide variety of ailments, including sore throats. Modern-day German studies show that ginger does kill viruses. "That's a lot more than most over-the-counter cough syrups or lozenges can do," says Allan Magaziner, D.O. "They only make you feel temporarily better, usually by numbing your throat to relieve pain."

Cut off a nickel-size piece of the fresh root, and just suck on it for 10 minutes, three times a day, until the infection is gone (one signal is that your mucus will be clear rather than yellow or green).

It's good for healing the *cause* of your pain, but Dr. Magaziner doesn't promise that ginger will bring immediate relief to severe pain. If your throat still hurts, alternate between ginger and hot tea or lozenges.

—**Allan Magaziner, D.O.,** *is the medical director of the Magaziner Center for Wellness and Anti-Aging Medicine in Cherry Hill, New Jersey, and author of* The Total Health Handbook.

WRAP YOURSELF IN COMFORT

When the flu gives you a stiff neck and achy shoulders, give it the hot towel treatment.

The flu can make shoulder muscles so tight that it hurts to lie down. When massage therapist Jennifer Dixon's son feels this way, she wraps him in a hot towel. Dixon finds that heat not only relaxes achy shoulders but also calms a cranky child (and surely a cranky grown-up, too).

Here's how to do a hot wrap: Wet a hand towel (a cloth slightly larger than a washcloth) and wring out the excess water. Roll it up, place it in a plastic bag, and then microwave it for 1 minute. The towel should be steaming when you remove it from the bag. When it feels cool enough to touch your skin, place it on the back of your shoulders and neck.

Lay a large dry bath towel on your bed (or wherever you would like to relax) and lie down. To lock in the heat around your upper back, wrap the ends of the dry towel that you are lying on around your shoulders. Cover up with blankets and relish the relief.

If you have a headache, add 2 drops of lavender essential oil to the hot towel. If you're congested, add 2 drops of eucalyptus essential oil. If you're experiencing both symptoms, drop both oils onto your towel.

Be careful not to get oils on the faces of infants and young children.

—Jennifer Dixon, C.M.T., *is a certified massage therapist and head of massage therapy at Amadeus Spa in Pasadena, California.*

CANCEL YOUR CHILLS WITH A SPICY SOAK

Sometimes even the thickest wool blankets and flannel pajamas can't keep you from shivering during a cold or flu outbreak. This is when it's time to take to the tub.

In Chinese medicine, a certain group of herbs are classified as "warming." These herbs increase circulation, which gives you a nice sensation of heating up, explains Ni Maishing, O.M.D., L.Ac.

When a cold brings chills, Dr. Maishing recommends getting into a hot tub with essential oils of the Asian warming herbs ginger, cinnamon, cardamom, and ylang-ylang. In addition to warming you up, studies show that this combination also works as a natural decongestant and helps the body re-sist the virus that started the chills.

Be sure that you don't substitute cinnamon bark oil for cinnamon leaf oil because the former is unsafe to apply to the skin.

Warming Oils

3 drops ginger essential oil
3 drops cinnamon leaf essential oil
5 drops cardamom essential oil
5 drops ylang-ylang essential oil
   Dab of shampoo

Fill your bath with hot water—as hot as you can handle. Stir the essential oils together with a quarter-size dab of shampoo in a small container (the shampoo acts as an emulsifier, allowing the essential oils to mix with the bathwater as opposed to floating on top of it). Add the mixture to your bathwater.

Climb into the tub and soak for about 15 minutes, but no longer than 20 minutes. After you get out of the tub, wrap yourself in towels. Then go to bed.

Do not use these oils for more than 2 weeks without the guidance of a qualified practitioner.

—Ni Maishing, O.M.D., L.Ac., *is a doctor of oriental medicine, acupuncturist, and director of the Union of Tao and Man Traditional Acupuncture in Santa Monica, California.*

MIX UP MOTHER NATURE'S COUGH SYRUP

When a cough or sore throat hits, reach in the pantry for sweet relief.

Cloves may add a piquant punch to desserts, but they also have merit as a pain reliever. Honey always adds a sweet touch not only to all sorts of food but also to the inflamed tissues of the throat. Together, they make a superbly soothing syrup, says Majid Ali, O.M.D., L.Ac.

While cloves dull throat pain, honey coats and moistens the throat—which should bring immediate relief to your discomfort, hoarseness, and coughing. Research from Germany shows that common cloves will also help your sore throat in the long run by destroying viruses and bacteria.

Combine 1 cup of honey and 5 or 6 whole cloves in a small container and refrigerate overnight. In the morning, strain out the cloves. Take 1 teaspoon to 1 tablespoon as needed. Refrigerate the syrup between use.

Because honey can contain traces of bacteria, don't give this remedy—or any product containing raw honey—to children under 2 years old.

—Majid Ali, O.M.D., L.Ac., *is a doctor of oriental medicine and licensed acupuncturist practicing complementary medicine in Los Angeles.*

PUT THE PRESSURE ON SINUS HEADACHES

Thanks to an ancient Chinese acupressure technique, it's easy to put an end to that throbbing across your forehead. Try your hand at this simple solution.

There isn't always an opportunity to make a break for an aspirin—say in the middle of a long-winded business meeting or waiting in the checkout line on the day before Thanksgiving. When you need quick relief without pills, acupressure is ideal.

Five thousand years ago, the Chinese recognized certain trigger points on the body that could be stimulated to relieve ailments. A point on the back of the hand in the angle between the forefinger and thumb is linked to the face and head. "Pressing a specific point in this area relieves the pressure

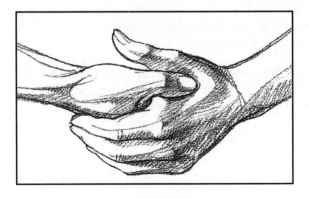

running from temple to temple during a sinus headache," says acupressurist Caroline Warner, C.M.T.

To find the correct pressure point, squeeze together the thumb and forefinger of your right hand. With your left hand, feel around for a tender spot in the top of the muscular hill that forms. When you've found the spot, release the thumb and forefinger of your right hand. Squeeze the pressure point with your left thumb on top and your forefinger on the palm. Sustain the pressure for 10 to 20 seconds, but not more than 30 seconds. Repeat the technique using your opposite hands the next time, until your headache goes away, adds Warner.

The headache-relieving effect isn't as long-lasting as aspirin, but it won't upset your stomach—and you won't lose your place in the checkout line.

—Caroline Warner, C.M.T., *is a certified massage therapist and an acupressure-massage therapist for crew and actors in* Jumanji *and other movie productions.*

DON'T DISCOUNT PILLOW POWER

Since "plenty of rest" is always the doctor's order, use a scented pillow to help soothe you to sleep.

A pillow stuffed with the grain hops is the perfect pampering accessory to break out when you're tossing and turning with the flu, because the grains massage your neck while emitting a sedating scent.

"If it helps you get to sleep, it's definitely worth trying. It's during sleep that our bodies' repair mechanisms are in full gear," says Bradley Bongiovanni, N.D. "All sorts of biochemical reactions take place while we are resting that allow for efficient recovery from illness."

Sleeping with hops pillows is reminiscent of a Victorian-era tradition to pamper or heal the body with herb- and grain-stuffed "dilly pillows." Dilly pillows might have marjoram leaves, for example, to relieve headaches, or evergreen needles and lemongrass to relieve *heart*aches for a weepy maiden.

But hops pillows are more than historic whimsy. One study showed that hops work directly on the nervous system to induce a sound sleep. Although the study tested hops internally, natural healers say that even *sniffing* the scent of hops has a sedative effect—especially as the hops age. Often, hops pillows also contain chamomile and lavender, which also have mildly tranquilizing scents.

Health food stores, yoga supply catalogs, and some pharmacies sell pillows made of hops that can help you snooze. You can make one for yourself or a friend by purchasing the hops from a health food store or bulk grain company.

—Bradley Bongiovanni, N.D., *is a naturopathic physician at Wellspace, a complementary health center in Cambridge, Massachusetts.*

SLATHER ON AN OATMEAL-MUSTARD PASTE

To clear up sinuses and stop back-of-the-throat dripping that causes a persistent cough, try an old-fashioned mustard poultice. The relief is worth the slippery-globby-gooiness.

A poultice is nothing more than a paste with crushed herbs applied directly to the skin. Although poultices may be time consuming to make and inevitably messy, this mustard poultice is so effective that it's worth the effort *and* worth making a little mess for, says holistic nurse Ellen Kamhi, R.N., Ph.D.

"Mustard increases circulation to the area where it is applied, which helps break up the secretions in the back of your throat," says Dr. Kamhi. Expect to feel a warm, tingling sensation when you apply this pack. That's the sign that the mustard is working its magic, she adds.

Because mustard is a strong herb, aloe vera is used in this recipe to protect the skin from mustard's natural irritants. Oatmeal not only provides the base for the paste but also contributes to the skin-soothing effect.

Chest Poultice

- 1   teaspoon powdered mustard
- ½   cup aloe vera gel
- ½   cup raw oatmeal
- 2–3 tablespoons hot water

Combine the ingredients using just enough water to make the mixture the consistency of thick breakfast oatmeal. When your poultice is cool enough to be comfortable to the skin, rub it all over your chest. Wrap gauze around your chest to keep the paste in place.

Climb into bed and place a warm washcloth on top of the mustard pack. Enjoy the sensation, leaving it on for about 20 minutes.

—Ellen Kamhi, R.N., Ph.D., *is a professional member of the American Herbalists Guild, author of* The Natural Medicine Chest, *and host of several national radio and television programs.*

LEAVE YOUR CONGESTION IN THE MIST

The classic humidifier is still one of the best remedies for chest congestion. Just don't let it backfire by breeding bacteria when you already have a cold to fight.

When congestion accompanies a cold, fire up the humidifier. "Water is the best expectorant for chest congestion. Adding it to the air helps loosen mucus and move it on its way," says pharmacist Donald Sullivan, R.Ph., Ph.D.

Dr. Sullivan uses a humidifier himself when he is feeling under the weather. But he is particular about how he uses it. "Mine is a cold water humidifier, not a hot water unit, which is much more prone to breeding bacteria," he says.

Set the cold water humidifier according to manufacturer's directions. To avoid mold in rugs and bedding, run the unit no more than 8 hours at a time. That means run it in your bedroom while you sleep and turn it off in the morning. Then empty the humidifier each morning to prevent bacteria from growing in the unit.

Stop using a humidifier once a cough becomes croupy (a hoarse cough). This is a sign that congestion is breaking up.

If you don't have a humidifier, try simmering a pot of water on the stove (just don't forget about it) or set a pot of water on the radiator or a flat hot-air vent.

—Donald Sullivan, R.Ph., Ph.D., *is a registered pharmacist; an assistant professor of pharmacy practice at Ohio Northern University College of Pharmacy in Ada, Ohio; and author of* A Senior's Guide to Healthy Travel.

MAKE YOUR OWN ROSE-MINT-LAVENDER COUGH DROPS

Asian medicine offers a delightful, gentle remedy for a hacking cough, based on some of America's most well-loved garden plants.

Need a break from those eye-watering lozenges from the pharmacy? This alternative to medicinal-tasting cough drops is tasty and truly sweet relief. Majid Ali, O.M.D., L.Ac., combines rose petal, mint, and lavender to create an all-natural cough drop.

These herbs are more than a pleasant combination for the palate. Rose petal breaks up congestion and blocks histamine, while mint cools the sting in your throat. Lavender actually retards pain signals to the brain. Honey moistens dry throats and has a slight antibacterial quality.

Use these cough drops as needed. They work for a dry or wet cough, says Dr. Ali. For variety, you could also combine the herbs with boiling water to create a soothing, fragrant tea.

Rose-Mint-Lavender Cough Drops

2–3   tablespoons dried rose petals
1–2   tablespoons fresh mint, diced
2–3   tablespoons dried lavender flowers
        About 2 teaspoons honey

Combine the herbs and grind them into a fine powder. Add enough honey to hold the herbs together. Divide the mixture into 12 equal portions and roll them into balls. Refrigerate the lozenges.

To avoid the chance of ingesting bacteria, don't give this remedy—or any product containing raw honey—to kids under 2 years of age.

—Majid Ali, O.M.D., L.Ac., *is a doctor of oriental medicine and licensed acupuncturist practicing complementary medicine in Los Angeles.*

SOCK COLD SYMPTOMS WITH WOOL POWER

If a stuffy chest is keeping you awake, then put on a pair of soggy socks, and believe it or not, you'll fall asleep breathing easy.

Climbing into bed with wet socks when you don't feel well may sound like the last thing you should do for a cold. But Bradley Bongiovanni, N.D., promotes this remedy to clear your head, throat, and chest—while bringing a host of other welcomed side effects.

A wet sock treatment can also relieve body aches and increase healing when you suffer from infections. Because it warms you up, it can also lull you into a relaxing sleep, says Dr. Bongiovanni.

Here's how it works: Blood stagnates in the area with the greatest congestion, which in this case is the upper body. Cold wet socks cause the blood vessels in the feet to constrict, which attracts the blood down toward the toes and thus away from your head, chest, and throat. Also, blood brings heat, which dry heavy socks trap in the area of your feet. This trapped heat dries the wet socks and warms you while you fall comfortably asleep.

Throwing on any old socks could cause you more harm than good because your feet won't dry out properly and you might have a chill all night. Be sure to follow Dr. Bongiovanni's prescription carefully.

Take a pair of cotton socks and dunk them in cold water. Be sure to wring out the socks thoroughly so they don't drip.

Warm your feet by soaking them in warm water for at least 10 to 15 minutes or taking a warm bath for 10 to 15 minutes. This step is very important. The treatment won't be as effective and could be harmful if your feet are not warmed first. Dry off your feet and body with a towel.

Place the cold wet socks (eek!) on your feet. Hurry and cover the cold socks with a second layer of the *dry* thick wool socks. Go directly to bed so you avoid getting chilled.

Keep the socks on overnight. You will find that the cotton socks will be dry in the morning and that your congestion will be reduced.

The wet sock treatment works best if repeated three nights in a row, adds Dr. Bongiovanni.

—Bradley Bongiovanni, N.D., *is a naturopathic physician at Wellspace, a complementary health center in Cambridge, Massachusetts.*

What to Eat and Drink

"Think of your cold as a cleansing process. The best thing you can do for yourself is to eat nutritious foods that have the power to boost immunity and encourage the elimination of germs."

—Elson M. Haas, M.D., *medical director of the Preventive Medical Center of Marin in San Rafael, California, and author of* Staying Healthy with Nutrition

53

DRINK YOUR WAY CLEAR

Consuming enough liquid is essential when you have a cold or flu. Noting the color of your urine will tell you whether you're properly quenched.

If your urine is highly concentrated and dark yellow, you're being way too stingy with liquid consumption. That's never good. But when you're ill, your body needs extra fluids to reduce congestion, fight fever, and aid your immune system. Sending lots of liquids into your body allows you to break up mucus and keep all your cells, including your immune cells, well-hydrated so they operate at their peak.

A good rule of thumb is to count the number of beverages you imbibe to insure you're getting adequate amounts, says Adria Sherman, Ph.D. At the bare minimum, pour yourself eight 8-ounce drinks per day. You'll know you're doing a good job when your urine is clear or light yellow.

Drinking water is best, because it doesn't contain unnecessary calories and sugars, Dr. Sherman says. Sports drinks are okay, too, but because their sodium content is high, she advises diluting them so they consist of half water. Caffeine has diuretic qualities, so sipping all day on coffee or caffeinated sodas will only work against you.

—Adria Sherman, Ph.D., *is a professor of nutritional sciences at Rutgers University in New Brunswick, New Jersey.*

Order the Light Fare

You've heard the adage, "Feed a cold, starve a fever." It turns out that avoiding solid food could be solid advice for some people, whether they have a cold or a fever.

Sneezing, coughing, and running a temperature are more than just uncomfortable symptoms—they're your body's way of trying to eliminate germs. Eating lightly or not at all is sometimes the best way to help the body do its job, advises Tori Hudson, N.D.

Liquids help keep phlegm moving out of the system, but solid foods just get in the way, creating more work in the digesting process. "Rather than put more in that your body has to deal with and metabolize, curb what's coming in," Dr. Hudson suggests.

Sticking solely to liquids won't work for everyone, however. A sudden fast could create a blood sugar crisis for people unaccustomed to light eating, or for anyone suffering from hypoglycemia or diabetes, Dr. Hudson warns. So if you must eat, choose a bowl of soup over a greasy hamburger, and avoid anything with lots of fats, proteins, and carbohydrates, which are difficult to digest.

If you do choose to forgo solid foods for a day or so, ladle out plenty of broth or thin soups for yourself, and drink diluted juices and caffeine-free teas to maintain your vitamin and fluid intake.

—Tori Hudson, N.D., *is a professor at the National College of Naturopathic Medicine and director of A Woman's Time naturopathic clinic in Portland, Oregon.*

FIGHT IT WITH FRUIT

Put fruit in your diet to help purge your body of cold and flu germs while boosting your immune response.

Elson M. Haas, M.D., encourages his patients to make good use of colds and flu bugs. The time you spend ailing is also the time to cleanse your body of germs, mucus, and other impurities. To do so, take advantage of the therapeutic value of fruit, he recommends.

Kiwifruit, grapefruit, oranges, tangerines, pineapples, and tropical fruits such as mangoes are all standouts on the cold-fighting front for two reasons. For one thing, they're chock-full of vitamin C, which is good for both diminishing cold symptoms and helping your immune system beat the virus. For another, juicy fruits have the liquids you need to wash toxins out of the body and loosen phlegm, while keeping you hydrated. Pineapples have an added benefit of aiding digestion.

Dr. Haas recommends eating a cocktail containing a wide variety of fruits when you have a cold. To treat your cold *and* your tastebuds, fix this pineapple fruit medley. If possible, use organically grown produce rather than chemically grown fruit, because your goal is to rid your body of impurities, and chemical residues will only make your immune system work harder.

Pineapple Fruit Medley

1¼ cups chopped pineapple
2 oranges, sectioned
2 tangerines, sectioned
3 kiwifruit, peeled and sliced
2 tablespoons lime juice

In a large bowl, combine the pineapple, oranges, tangerines, and kiwifruit. Drizzle with lime juice. Cover and allow to marinate in the refrigerator for 1 hour.

For a truly cleansing diet, Dr. Haas suggests sticking strictly to fruit salads and vegetable soups, eaten at separate meals for several days.

—**Elson M. Haas, M.D.,** *is the founder and medical director of the Preventive Medical Center of Marin in San Rafael, California, and author of* Staying Healthy with Nutrition.

BEAT COLDS WITH BELL PEPPERS

You don't have to overload on traditional citrus to get a blast of vitamin C. Bell peppers are loaded with this tried-and-true, super-cold-whopping nutrient.

Since ascorbic acid researcher Linus Pauling's time, reams of research have stacked up showing that vitamin C can reduce the length and severity of colds. What's more, it's believed to be capable of decreasing inflammation of the nasal passages.

Eating bell peppers is a marvelous way to increase your daily intake of this beneficial vitamin, says nutrition researcher Carol S. Johnston, Ph.D. Other vegetables such as broccoli and cauliflower are good, too, but bell peppers top even those. The C content in a single yellow pepper totals a walloping 350 milligrams, while red peppers hold 225 and green peppers pack 106 milligrams of vitamin C.

Pauling was known to supplement daily with 8,000 milligrams of vitamin C. While that much could be excessive, it's essential to consume several C-rich foods throughout the day. Vitamin C is considered a water-soluble vitamin, which means your body doesn't retain it for very long. (Dr. Johnston takes in 2,000 milligrams when she feels a cold coming on.)

Oranges and grapefruit provide a good breakfast C supply, but try working bell peppers into your lunch and dinner, Dr. Johnston advises. Eating peppers raw will guarantee the most vitamin C, but heating them also releases another tremendous cold-combating antioxidant, beta-carotene.

If you have to work while you have a cold, bring the following easy casserole for lunch. It contains both red peppers and tomatoes to supply you with plenty of cold-combating C, and it's brimming with other immune-boosting nutrients as well. Don't fret about the little bit of fat in the oil—it's needed to help you absorb vitamins into the bloodstream.

Bulgur and Sweet Pepper Lunch Casserole

½   cup stock
½   cup bulgur
3   garlic cloves, minced
4   plum tomatoes, chopped
2   sweet red peppers, julienned
¼   cup apple cider vinegar
1   tablespoon olive oil
½   teaspoon dried thyme
1   teaspoon snipped chives

In a 1-quart saucepan, bring the stock to a boil. Add the bulgur and garlic. Cover, remove from heat (bulgur does not have to cook), and let stand for 20 minutes or until the liquid has been absorbed. Fluff with a fork and place in a large bowl.

(continued)

Add the tomatoes and peppers. Toss to combine.

In a cup, whisk together the vinegar, oil, thyme, and chives. Pour over the bulgur. Toss to combine.

This dish can be eaten cold or hot.

Makes 4 servings.

—Carol S. Johnston, Ph.D., *is an associate professor of food and nutrition in the department of family resources at the Arizona State University in Tempe.*

DON'T DO DAIRY

Although a numbing scoop of ice cream might sound like the perfect salve for a scratchy throat, it might just make matters worse.

Ice cream, like all dairy products, should be avoided when your nose starts running, says Martha H. Howard, M.D. Milk can actually stimulate the production of mucus—obviously not a desirable outcome if you're already blowing through tissues by the boxful.

Just why dairy products—including milk, cheese, creamy sauces, and desserts—create mucus isn't clear, Dr. Howard notes. It could be caused by an allergic reaction to milk proteins or milk sugar (lactose). And in the case of commercial milk, the presence of pesticides, antibiotics, and growth hormones could potentially cause allergic reactions. But studies show that dairy products are mucus forming even in people not allergic to milk, she explains.

Most people notice that they have to clear their throats after a glass of milk or a slice of cheese. That's because they feel the mucus buildup, Dr. Howard says. When you have a cold, that additional mucus is the last thing you need. Not only is it uncomfortable but it also can lead to sinus blockage, possibly promoting secondary infections.

"The more mucus you have, the more clogged your sinuses can become, and then you can have both a sinus infection *and* a cold," says Dr. Howard.

—Martha H. Howard, M.D., *is a Chinese medicine specialist and medical director of Wellness Associates of Chicago.*

MIX UP SOME MOONGDAL

According to traditional Indian medicine, when you have a cold, you need to build "a central digestive fire" in order to overcome an imbalance of the energies in the body. In western terms, that means eat what's easy to digest.

Ayurvedic medicine perceives disease as a result of toxins, and toxins are usually the result of undigested, unabsorbed, or unassimilated food. Congestion is caused by *kapha,* the force inside you that creates structure and solidity.

So when kapha accumulates anywhere, including the respiratory system, it's necessary to cater to your digestive system so you can eliminate impurities and get energy moving again, explains Ayurvedic doctor Jay L. Glaser, M.D.

Once you free up kapha, you'll lose that achy, tired, tight feeling. To get back in balance, eat lightly of fresh foods that are simple to digest during a cold outbreak—something that western doctors also endorse.

Dr. Glaser recommends preparing moongdal soup, a dish made of mung beans and spices. The small, dried green beans are available in health food stores and some groceries.

Moongdal soup is tasty, and it's beneficial because all the ingredients aid digestion, says Dr. Glaser.

Moongdal Soup

½	cup dried mung beans
6	cups water
5	slices (nickel-size) fresh gingerroot
1–2	teaspoons turmeric
	Cumin
	Salt
	Black pepper

Mix the beans with the water. Add the fresh gingerroot and turmeric, plus cumin, salt, and black pepper to taste. Bring to a boil and let simmer, covered, about 1 hour, or until a thick soup is formed. Eat the soup for your main meal, along with small amounts of steamed, fresh vegetables such as zucchini, green beans, or spinach.

—Jay L. Glaser, M.D., *is the medical director of the Maharishi Ayurvedic Health Center in Lancaster, Massachusetts.*

OUST IT WITH ONIONS

If you've been raised on cherry-tasting cough syrup, this is going to take some getting used to. But once you can get over the shock of "onion medicine," your respiratory tract will thank you.

You might have thought about them only as the star ingredient in cheesy French soup and the zing in potato salad. Actually, onions have medicinal value, too. They act as an expectorant, loosening up mucus that's trapped in nasal or bronchial passages. When you have a dry, irritating cough, eating onions can help ease phlegm so you can cough it out. Onions are also antiviral, which means they offer the long-term benefit of helping you overcome the virus causing your cold and flu.

An old folk remedy calls for taking advantage of the onion's expectorant qualities by cooking it with some throat-soothing honey. "It makes a great cough syrup," says herbal expert David Winston. Here's a recipe Winston recommends.

Onion Cough Syrup

    6 medium onions
    1 cup honey
    1 cup water

In a large baking pan, combine the onions, honey, and water. Bake in an oven heated to 325°F for 1 to 1½ hours, or until the onions fall apart. While they're still hot, remove the onions and squeeze them through a strainer so that the juice drips back into the syrup. Take 1 tablespoon at a time, as needed.

—David Winston *is the president of Herbalist and Alchemist Inc., a school and herbal medicine company in Washington, New Jersey, and a founding member of the American Herbalists Guild.*

SPICE UP YOUR MENU

Capsaicin is the chemical that puts the heat into hot peppers. It's also a natural decongestant, capable of bringing instant relief to stuffy heads and dry coughs.

If you think spicy salsa and hot sauce are only condiments for Mexican feasts, think again. A little bit of a hot-pepper product can unstuff noses, clear bronchial tubes, and lubricate dry throats, says Varro E. Tyler, Ph.D., Sc.D.

What's the best way to serve up this spicy tonic? Buy dried red pepper flakes and sprinkle them into foods, Dr. Tyler recommends. Tabasco sauce will also do the job. There's no formula for figuring how much to add. Because sensitivity to spicy foods varies, you should adjust pepper quantities to your own tolerance, says Dr. Tyler.

Even small amounts will bring immediate relief. But keep your spices handy. Those sinuses won't stay clear too long, so you'll have to pep up soups, stews, salads, or stir-fries several times a day.

—Varro E. Tyler, Ph.D., Sc.D., *is distinguished professor emeritus of pharmacognosy at Purdue University in West Lafayette, Indiana, and author of* Tyler's Honest Herbal.

DRINK YOUR CARROTS

Your body needs a good supply of vitamins and minerals as well as extra liquid when it's battling a cold, and vegetables deliver the right stuff.

When it comes to vitamins, reaching for your juicer is a lot better than reaching for your supplements, according to Andrea D. Sullivan, N.D., Ph.D. With supplements, it's not known how much is absorbed into the body. "In food form, your body usually processes vitamins more completely," she explains.

Vegetable juice gives you vitamins in concentrated amounts, says Dr. Sullivan. One of the best drinks you can make when you have a cold or flu is carrot juice. It's rich in beta-carotene, which helps keep the immune system in good working order. To fix yourself a truly vitamin-powered drink, blend carrots with other vegetables.

One cold- and flu-busting drink combo that Dr. Sullivan recommends is carrot, beet, and celery juice. Carrots should comprise about half the mixture, and the other ingredients about one-fourth each. Add water to taste. Use beets sparingly, because they contain sugar, which hampers the immune system, says Dr. Sullivan. If you make carrot juice alone, dilute it with about ¼ cup water. All juices should be prepared using a juicer—it needn't be expensive, and recipes are usually included.

—Andrea D. Sullivan, N.D., Ph.D., *is a naturopathic and homeopathic physician in Washington, D.C., and author of* A Path to Healing.

CHICKEN SOUP WITH A TWIST

Chicken soup is the classic cure for a cold. But to maximize its healing effect, take a tip from the ancient Egyptians— add fresh lemon juice to the pot.

American caretakers have long served chicken soup to pamper the bedridden, and modern doctors have acknowledged the soup's true healing virtues. Researchers at Mount Sinai Medical Center in Miami Beach concluded that the broth in chicken soup increases the flow of mucus and shortens the time that cold germs spend inside the nose. And it's no surprise that pharmacists created a drug to treat bronchitis and respiratory infections using an amino acid found in chickens.

Better yet, there's one ingredient that can add extra healing power, says Katherine D. Sherif, M.D. "My Egyptian grandmother squeezed a whole lemon into a pot of fresh chicken soup."

In Egypt, where cold sufferers also drink fresh lemonade throughout the day, lemons are extolled as great cold busters. As citrus fruits, lemons are packed with immune-supportive vitamin C. What's more, some doctors recommend lemons for their natural astringent properties, which stimulate the liver and encourage your body to flush out germs.

For the most nourishing soup, start from scratch with a whole chicken that simmers until the juices are no longer pink. Add your favorite ingredients—carrots, celery, garlic, and onions will bestow flavor and vitamins. Just before serving, squeeze in the juice of one lemon.

—Katherine D. Sherif, M.D., *is an assistant professor in the department of medicine at M.C.P. Hahnemann University in Philadelphia.*

SIP SOME
SOUTH AMERICAN TEA

Can't face the prospect of 7 days sniffling and sneezing? The solution might be growing in the soil of Argentina, Brazil, and Paraguay.

In South America, they send colds packing by guzzling lots and lots of a concentrated tea made from the traditional plants yerba mate and lapacho. Plant therapy researcher Daniel B. Mowrey, Ph.D., says the stuff really works.

High in vitamins C and A and packed with pantothenic acid (an essential B vitamin), the drink kicks the immune system into high gear, Dr. Mowrey explains. He suggests drinking 2 quarts a day for several days whenever you have a cold.

Lapacho, the bark of a jungle tree, is also known as Pau d'Arco or taheebo. Yerba mate is roasted leaves from a South American holly tree. Both plants can be purchased at health food stores and through herb company catalogs.

Begin with a strong concoction that's made by pouring 12 heaping tablespoons of the loose tea—that's 6 each of yerba mate leaves and lapacho bark—into 1 quart of hot water. If you prefer iced tea, it's not necessary to brew in boiling water, although this elixir is somewhat more effective hot. Strain the solids and set aside, and sip the tea throughout the day. Later, add the strainings to a second quart of water to make a weaker infusion, and drink that throughout the evening.

This tea should not be taken during pregnancy, but otherwise it presents no adverse side effects for short-term use. Just be aware that yerba mate contains small amounts of caffeine.

Be savvy when buying lapacho, Dr. Mowrey warns. The only part of the plant that is therapeutic is the inner lining of the bark, so look for a thin, papery substance, not woody chunks.

—Daniel B. Mowrey, Ph.D., *is the president of the American Phytotherapy Research Laboratory in Salt Lake City and author of* The Scientific Validation of Herbal Medicine.

DON'T HYDRATE WITH HIGH-SUGAR DRINKS

Drinking lots of fluids makes sense when you have a cold or flu, but sipping sugary soft drinks and fruit juices can be counterproductive. Sugar can work to deplete your body of necessary fluids.

Downing tall glasses of fruit juice might seem like a judicious way to treat a cold. Not so, says Katherine D. Sherif, M.D. When you're fighting a cold or flu, avoid anything high in sugar, including fruit juices, she recommends.

Drinks that have high sugar concentration act as diuretics, which means they force from your body the very fluids you need to stay hydrated when you're sick. "When you're dried out, your white blood cells don't work as well," Dr. Sherif explains. And when you lose those fluids, you also lose vitamins and nutrients you'd be better off retaining.

To get the best benefit from your beverages, choose ones that aren't sweet. Water and seltzer water are both preferable. If you crave soft drinks, grab a diet soda, but you're much better off swallowing liquids with other nutritional gains. Soups, for example, can provide you with valuable vitamins and proteins. Herbal teas, such as chamomile, offer an added bonus of relaxing as well as hydrating you. But leave caffeinated teas and coffee on the shelf, since caffeine also has a diuretic effect.

—Katherine D. Sherif, M.D., *is an assistant professor in the department of medicine at M.C.P. Hahnemann University in Philadelphia.*

SOOTHE IT SAGELY

Don't let sage just sit in your spice rack until Thanksgiving rolls around. Taking it when you have a cold or a scratchy throat is a wise idea.

Sage is one of the best herbs around when it comes to relieving a sore throat. It not only soothes the pain but also has antiviral and antibacterial qualities, and it's an antioxidant to boot, says herbal expert David Winston. All that "anti" adds up to a big plus when you're miserable, because it means sage helps oust infections, while the antioxidants aid immune cells.

You can add sage to your diet by sprinkling the dried flakes into foods. As with most herbs, though, if you cook it heavily, you will destroy its therapeutic value. Adding sage at the end of cooking, just before serving, allows it to retain its germ-fighting abilities.

To fix a sore throat, sage is best served as a tea, says Winston. To prepare, pour 8 ounces of boiling water into a mug. Add 1 to 2 teaspoons of dried sage, cover, and allow to steep 20 to 30 minutes. Winston recommends drinking a 4-ounce cupful four times a day for maximum benefits. How does it taste? Pretty intense, says Winston. "But it works nicely," he adds. To improve flavor, add honey and lemon to taste.

This tea is not recommended for pregnant women.

—**David Winston** *is the president of Herbalist and Alchemist Inc., a school and herbal medicine company in Washington, New Jersey, and a founding member of the American Herbalists Guild.*

GIVE YOUR THROAT THE GOLD TREATMENT

People whose moms served them tea with honey after playing too long in the snow know that this sweetener is golden for easing sore throat pain. It might also help you heal faster.

Honey has been part of humankind's pharmacopoeia since ancient Egyptian and Grecian times, when it was used for everything from burns to surgery. Today, honey still has a place in the medicine chest, says Adriane Fugh-Berman, M.D.

A study conducted at Hebrew University in Jerusalem found that honey can do more than temporarily take the "ow" out of your swallow. Researchers tested volunteers to determine the effect of honey on salivary bacteria. The results: Bacteria counts dropped following a concentrated application of honey and remained low for 1 hour afterward.

"In medical school we experimented with killing bacteria by dropping honey on it," Dr. Fugh-Berman says. "While oral bacteria occurs normally, lowering bacteria counts when you have a cold or flu could possibly help your body stave off infection."

Another healing boost the sweet medicine offers is a dose of nutrients that include vitamin C and a range of B vitamins. According to studies, darker honeys contain more vitamins than lighter ones.

Taking a teaspoon every few hours while your throat is tender could possibly provide resistance to the virus that causes sore throats, while also offering sweet relief, Dr. Fugh-Berman adds.

—Adriane Fugh-Berman, M.D., *is an assistant clinical professor at George Washington University School of Medicine in Washington, D.C. and the chairperson of the National Women's Health Network.*

HOLD THE ICE

Traditional Chinese medicine agrees with western practices when it comes to treating colds and flu with plenty of fluids. But Chinese doctors would never serve their patients a cold drink.

Hot and room-temperature liquids are a staple of tradi-tional Chinese cold therapy, but chilled juices and ice water are off limits. So are foods fresh out of the refrigerator. That's because when you swallow something cold, it's a shock to your respiratory and digestive systems, says Martha H. Howard, M.D.

Any part of your body that comes in contact with a cold food or liquid has to work to get warm again, Dr. Howard ex-plains. It takes energy to bring the affected cells back to room temperature, and that detracts from the energy that's available to help your body heal.

Lukewarm or hot liquids, on the other hand, moisturize the throat and encourage your system to digest food prop-erly, flush out the cold virus, and thin mucus secretions. Therefore, Chinese medicine calls for drinking very weak black or green teas or, more traditionally, hot water with no tea added. And all food or drinks are served at room tem-perature or warmer, except in very hot weather, and even then iced drinks are avoided.

—Martha H. Howard, M.D., *is a Chinese medicine specialist and medical director of Wellness Associates of Chicago.*

THE PROOF IS IN THE PORRIDGE

Maybe the three bears were out taking a brisk walk first thing in the morning because they got their stamina from this stuff. It can also make you well when you're under the weather.

Goldilocks didn't know how smart the wooly family she visited actually was. Rice porridge is a centuries-old breakfast tradition, which the Chinese knew could supply a lot of energy—vital when you're fighting a cold, says Majid Ali, O.M.D., L.Ac. With some "doctoring," this cereal can also cool fevers and fight infections.

"In Chinese medicine, illnesses are considered 'cold' or 'hot' and are treated with herbs of opposing temperatures," says Dr. Ali. "Therefore, if a cold causes chills, we use warming herbs like garlic, ginger, and hot pepper. When the flu causes a fever, we cool it with mint and parsley."

Here is Dr. Ali's standard porridge with adaptations for specific symptoms.

Rice Porridge for Colds and Flu

½ cup rice (or package of cream of rice cereal)
2½ cups water

For Colds

1 tablespoon freshly grated gingerroot
2 garlic cloves, crushed
2–3 drops hot sauce (optional)

(continued)

For Flu

2 teaspoons fresh mint, finely chopped (or 1 teaspoon dried)

1 teaspoon fresh parsley, finely chopped (or ½ teaspoon dried)

Combine the rice and water in a small saucepan. Cover and bring to a boil. Lower the heat and let simmer for about 15 minutes. Remove the porridge from the heat and add the appropriate herbs and spices, depending on whether you need to warm up or cool down.

—Majid Ali, O.M.D., L.Ac., *is a doctor of oriental medicine and licensed acupuncturist practicing complementary medicine in Los Angeles.*

LICK THAT COUGH WITH LICORICE

If you like this plant's taste, it's a pleasant way of getting your medicine. When stirred into a tea, powdered licorice root soothes dry throats and halts coughs for hours.

Dry, hacking coughs or pesky tickles can rankle the already troubled cold sufferer. But sweet relief is only a sip away. Licorice tea has an expectorant effect that can quiet coughs and relieve dry throats, says Varro E. Tyler, Ph.D., Sc.D. It works by stimulating secretions in the mucous membranes, and that helps ease phlegm. Once phlegm starts moving, the throat feels moister and coughs loosen up.

Dr. Tyler recommends mixing 1 teaspoon of powdered licorice root into a cup of hot water for a concoction that will keep your throat clear for several hours. Licorice cough drops are also effective, but licorice candy probably won't do the trick. Most American-made licorice candy is flavored with anise and contains no real licorice root, explains Dr. Tyler.

Licorice teas can be repeated three times a day, but not for more than a week and never in large quantities, says Dr. Tyler. Overuse can lead to water retention, high blood pressure caused by potassium loss, or damage to the heart and kidneys. And don't use this remedy if you have diabetes, high blood pressure, liver or kidney disorders, or low potassium levels.

—Varro E. Tyler, Ph.D., Sc.D., *is distinguished professor emeritus of pharmacognosy at Purdue University in West Lafayette, Indiana, and author of* Tyler's Honest Herbal.

PUT PASTE IN THE POT

The fermented soy paste, miso, has been a staple in the Japanese diet for more than 2,500 years. It's the star ingredient in the eastern world's answer to chicken soup.

Vegetable soups are essential when you have a cold or flu. They keep the bodily fluids from the nasal passages thin enough to spit or blow them out, while providing a wallop of vitamins," says Tori Hudson, N.D. Miso paste brings additional antioxidants that support the immune system by protecting cells from damage.

What's more, miso paste settles the stomach, so it's a wise choice when the flu leaves you feeling nauseated.

Miso is available in several varieties from health food stores and Asian groceries. The traditional Japanese paste is always made from fermented soy beans but can also be flavored with other grains, which will alter the color and flavor. The yellow-colored varieties are buttery-tasting and less salty than smoky-flavored dark misos.

In fact, the pale-colored garbanzo and millet misos—for you traditionalists—actually taste similar to chicken broth. If you are new to miso, start off with a milder, light variety.

Simple Miso Soup

3 cups low-sodium vegetable or mushroom stock
3 cups water
   Miso, to taste
1 cup thinly sliced carrot sticks
1 cup coarsely chopped spinach
1 cup thinly sliced sweet red peppers
1 cup cubed extra-firm tofu
1 teaspoon minced fresh gingerroot
1 tablespoon toasted sesame seeds

In a 3-quart saucepan over medium-high heat, bring the stock and water to a boil. Ladle out ¼ cup of the liquid and place it in a cup. Add the miso (the more miso you add, the richer and saltier the soup will be) and mix well to dissolve it. Set aside.

Reduce the heat to medium. Stir in the carrots. After 1 minute, add the spinach, peppers, tofu, and gingerroot. Cook until the vegetables are tender, or about 5 minutes.

Just before serving, add the miso mixture. (Don't boil the miso or you will destroy the enzymes that are beneficial to your digestion.) Simmer for 2 minutes. Sprinkle with sesame seeds before serving.

Makes 4 servings.

—Tori Hudson, N.D., *is a professor at the National College of Naturopathic Medicine and director of A Woman's Time naturopathic clinic in Portland, Oregon.*

Letting Nature Take Its Course

"If you want to get better quicker, the key is to stimulate the incredible healing power within the body rather than trying to suppress and control symptoms."

—Bradley Bongiovanni, N.D.,
*naturopathic physician at Wellspace,
a complementary health center in
Cambridge, Massachusetts*

BREAK A FEVER WITH BONESET

Boneset is an herb that promotes sweating to allow your fever to run its course quickly and effectively.

Unlike aspirin, which artificially brings down the body temperature so you don't feel so hot, fever-treatment herbs actually make you sweat. This is not as peculiar as it sounds, says Rena Bloom, N.D.

Taking aspirin might make you *feel* more comfortable temporarily, but remember this: Aspirin doesn't help fight the infection or cure the disease. By using herbs instead, your fever spikes to a higher reading (102°F is ideal), you go through a sweaty period called *flush,* and then the whole thing should be over with.

You might feel worse temporarily before you feel better, but in the long run you let your fever run its course—which helps your body work at its best to overcome the flu naturally.

Fevers that get close to 106°F are dangerous, however, not to mention excruciating. So if your fever starts to spike over 104°F, you can lower it naturally by taking a cool bath. If it stays higher than 104°F or lasts for more than 2 days, see a doctor.

Boneset tea is one sweat-promoting herb that Dr. Bloom recommends. The only problem with boneset is its bitter taste, but honey can make it more pleasant.

Use 1 tablespoon of dried boneset per cup of boiling water and let it steep for 10 minutes, then add honey to taste. Drink it three times a day.

If you're prone to allergies—particularly to chamomile, feverfew, ragweed, or other members of the daisy family—you might also have an allergic reaction to boneset. It's important to take no more than the recommended amount. (Boneset can cause vomiting and diarrhea when ingested in large doses.)

—**Rena Bloom, N.D.,** *is a naturopathic physician practicing in Denver.*

RUB YOUR CHEST WITH ONIONS

Onions are more than a topping for burgers and salads. Putting them on top of your chest is actually a natural method of reducing congestion and fighting infection.

This culinary staple has a much more noble role than as a flavor enhancer. Among herbalists, the onion is highly valued for reducing flu and cold symptoms, and there are legitimate reasons for its popularity, says herbal expert Feather Jones.

When cut, onions emit an oil that has virus-fighting properties. Because this oil (the same one that makes you tear) works as a natural vasodilator, causing your pores to open, you get the oils into your lungs by laying cut onions on your chest.

In this remedy you'll add heat, which also opens pores, causing the healing oil to penetrate deeper into the chest. Another benefit is that the heat causes increased circulation in your chest, which breaks up congestion.

Jones recommends taking one large or two small onions and coarsely dicing them. Place the pieces in a pan and sauté them with a little oil until they are transparent. Let them cool, and then lay them across your chest. Cover with a piece of plastic wrap large enough to overlap the onions by 1 inch. Then lay a hot water bottle or a warm towel on top. Leave the onions in place about half an hour, she says.

—Feather Jones *is a professional member of the American Herbalists Guild and director of the Rocky Mountain Center for Botanical Studies in Boulder, Colorado.*

OIL AWAY YOUR FLU

Rub down with a stimulating mix of essential oils and feel your flu symptoms diminish.

At the first sign of flu symptoms, boost your immune defenses by trying a blend of essential oils recommended by licensed massage therapist Susanne Wissell: ravensara, eucalyptus, and cinnamon leaf.

The essential oil ravensara contributes congestion relief to the formula. Eucalyptus is an antibacterial and antiviral oil. Cinnamon leaf also has anti-infection properties, she adds. Be sure that you don't substitute cinnamon bark oil for cinnamon leaf oil because the former is unsafe to apply to the skin.

Essential Oil Flu Rub

1   ounce vegetable or almond oil
11 drops eucalyptus essential oil
11 drops ravensara essential oil
2   drops cinnamon leaf oil

In a small container, combine the vegetable or almond oil and the essential oils. Thoroughly mix the solution, using a dropper to stir it. Then, using your hands, rub the oils on your throat and upper chest area.

Don an old pair of pajamas that you don't mind getting some oil on, and apply this treatment several times throughout the day, suggests Wissell. Then apply it again at bedtime. For maximum effect, combine this oil treatment with Ginger and Garlic Tea (see page 96). "Don't be surprised if by the next morning you feel like a new person," Wissell says.

You can continue this treatment until all the symptoms subside, but not longer than 2 weeks. (By this time your flu should be gone. If not, seek medical treatment.)

—Susanne Wissell, L.M.T., *is a licensed massage therapist and principal of the Center for Holistic Botanical Studies in Wakefield, Massachusetts.*

WATER DOWN CONGESTION WITH HYDROTHERAPY

Using water to treat illness dates back to Hippocrates in the fourth century B.C. This particular method works by increasing circulation throughout the respiratory system.

Lymph, the bodily fluid that collects in your glands, is rich in disease-destroying white blood cells. When your glands are swollen, it's a good sign that you have lots of lymph at work, putting up a good fight against your cold or flu virus. By applying cold water and a warming scarf to your neck, you are using hydrotherapy to maximize the defense mechanisms already in place through blood and lymph flow, says Nancy Dunne Boggs, N.D.

First, warm up your skin by taking a quick warm bath or shower. Before your throat cools, soak a cotton bandana with cold water, wring it out well, and wrap it comfortably around your throat. Quickly cover the wet cotton with a dry wool scarf, tying it securely, but not too tightly, around your neck. Then get right into bed. You should feel relaxing refreshment in less than a minute after settling under the warm covers, Dr. Boggs says.

Why does it work? The cold water causes blood vessels at the surface of your skin to narrow, so blood and lymph retreat to deeper tissue. The whole area heats up from the activity of blood and lymph fluid. The wool retains the heat, soon causing you to sweat. The heating and then cooling off on the surface from perspiration stimulates another flush of blood and lymph through the respiratory system, and the cycle repeats itself.

Ultimately, any congesting fluid in the throat, sinuses, and middle ear is drained by the movement of blood and lymph, while the virus is being fought by increased immune cell activity, adds Dr. Boggs.

You should sleep very comfortably, but Dr. Boggs recommends that you keep the wrap on for at least 2 hours. Leaving the bandana and scarf on all night is fine.

—Nancy Dunne Boggs, N.D., *is a naturopathic physician practicing in Missoula, Montana, and founder of Bitterroot Natural Medicine, a botanical products company.*

DON'T OVERDO NOSE SPRAYS

Spray your stuffy nose too often, and you'll be spraying away your natural protection against more serious conditions like sinusitis.

Over-the-counter medicated nose sprays sometimes cause more harm than good. For starters, they interfere with one of the body's most clever defense mechanisms.

When your body realizes that a cold or flu bug is intruding, it reacts by flooding the thousands of tiny blood vessels in the nose with blood, causing the membranes to swell. This makes it more difficult for invaders to travel further into the body. At the same time, the body releases its germ-fighting white cells in a stream of mucus, in an attempt to search out and destroy these invaders, says Gailen D. Marshall Jr., M.D., Ph.D.

In addition to interfering with this protective feature,

nasal sprays can damage the cell linings of the nose's mucosal tissue by causing them to lose their microscopic hairs (cilia), which are crucial for keeping the normal mucus coating in the nose working smoothly. Dr. Marshall warns that, in the long run, overuse could lead to recurrent sinus infections.

If you must use a decongestant spray, use it no more than twice a day for a maximum of 3 or 4 days in a row. Then take an equal amount of time off. Over-the-counter nasal spray decongestants are among the most potentially addictive of all drugs, Dr. Marshall says. When you notice that its effectiveness lasts for a shorter time, there's a good chance you're becoming dependent on it, and it's time to stop.

Safer options are the natural decongestants discussed here and in Soothing Healers on page 31 and What to Eat and Drink on page 53.

—Gailen D. Marshall Jr., M.D., Ph.D., *is an associate professor and director of the Allergy and Clinical Immunology Division at the University of Texas Medical School in Houston.*

TREAT A STUFFY NOSE WITH TABASCO

Tabasco gives a Bloody Mary its zing, but did you know it could also break your cold and flu congestion? Here are a few hot tips to help your stuffy nose.

True, the mucus that your body produces when you're sick helps prevent the spread of a cold virus, and a runny nose carries out germs. But however benevolent they might be, these symptoms are still annoying.

Hot spices and peppers are a solution to kick the self-cleaning process into high gear—so nature can *really* run its course, says Nancy Dunne Boggs, N.D.

Because hot spices make your nose run, they thin out mucus, quickly clearing clogged nasal passages—without disrupting the body's natural defenses. Dr. Boggs recommends a good homemade tonic for this purpose.

Spicy Congestion Tonic

      Juice of ½ lemon
    1 teaspoon honey
    ⅛ teaspoon ground cayenne pepper
    8 ounces hot water

Add the lemon, honey, and pepper to the water. Have this drink two or three times a day until your symptoms diminish. Lemon has astringent properties that also help the body flush out germs, and the honey is for flavor.

You can also use hot pepper sauce. Just shake the bottle well, put 10 drops of that red fire into 8 ounces of water, and drink up. Do this three times a day for as long as you have symptoms, she says. You can increase the hot sauce to 20 drops to ease congestion, but cut back to 10 drops if your stomach starts burning.

—Nancy Dunne Boggs, N.D., *is a naturopathic physician practicing in Missoula, Montana, and founder of Bitterroot Natural Medicine, a botanical products company.*

PUT THE SQUEEZE ON LINGERING COLDS WITH ACUPRESSURE

Follow this sequence of acupressure techniques to help your body better fight and feel relief from a variety of cold symptoms.

Chinese doctors have known for more than 5,000 years that stimulating certain acupressure points on the body can the bring relief from the symptoms of a cold. Now you can try your hand at this ancient method with the following sequence of healing touches.

If you feel unbearable pain when stimulating any of these points, you're probably pressing too hard; but tenderness means you have probably found the correct place, says acupressure practitioner Michael Reed Gach, Ph.D. Stimulate each point for 1 minute.

This is a sequence for relieving general cold symptoms, especially congestion. Starting with K27, press your thumbs into both points in the hollows below the head of your collar bone, firmly and steadily, while breathing slowly. Move to GB20, under the base of your skull, and press both points with your thumbs, deeply (your other fingers are gently cradling your head). Then move to LI11, in the hollow at the end of your elbow. Stimulate this point with the middle finger of your opposite hand for 1 minute before doing the same with the opposite elbow and middle finger. Then return to K27 and repeat the entire sequence.

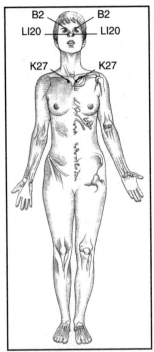

**Pressure Points
(Front View)**

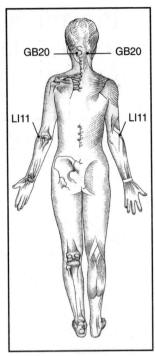

**Pressure Points
(Back View)**

This should be done at least three times a day for maximum relief. "Because acupressure balances your body to expel the virus more quickly, it might seem that your cold is temporarily worsening. The body is simply progressing through the symptoms faster than usual," Dr. Gach says.

For sniffly, sneezy symptoms in particular, Dr. Gach recommends 1 minute of pressure on both of the following points: Press your middle and index fingers on your face just beside both nostrils, pressing up and underneath the cheekbones (LI20); then press your thumbs in the upper ridges of the eye sockets, close to the bridge of the nose (B2).

—Michael Reed Gach, Ph.D., *is the director of the Acupressure Institute in Berkeley, California, and author of* Acupressure's Potent Points.

TRY THE YOGA ALTERNATIVE TO NASAL SPRAYS

A nasal lavage is a yoga tradition that can relieve congestion and help you avoid sinus infections. But it has nothing to do with stretching or contorting your body.

If you can stand the side effects, over-the-counter decongestants usually do reduce nasal congestion—but only for a short period of time. Unfortunately, when you stop, your symptoms are still there, or they become worse, says Bradley Bongiovanni, N.D.

A salt water nasal lavage, which is nothing more than washing out your sinuses, actually improves the tone of your sinuses—so you can feel better longer, and your long-term defenses are strengthened.

These are the supplies you'll need.

- Salt—sea salt is best
- 2 ounces of filtered or bottled water
- A towel or washcloth
- A workable container—yoga supply catalogs and Ayurvedic medicine shops sell a specially designed pot, a

neti pot, which has a spout that fits comfortably in one nostril. Other tools that work include a clean turkey baster, bulb syringe, or small watering pot.

Here's how to proceed: Thoroughly dissolve 1 teaspoon of salt into approximately 2 cups of warm water, and fill your container. Then insert the spout into one nostril as you lean over a sink. Imagine pointing the very top of your head toward the faucet, then tilting slightly to the side, opposite to where the spout is inserted.

The idea is to run the salt water up one nostril and out the other, while breathing through your mouth. You will feel the water move into the right nostril and exit the left. Do this until you have used up about a cup of water. Then use the rest of the solution on the other side. It's fine that some of the water drains into your mouth—just spit it out.

When the water is used up, expel the water trapped in your nose by blowing out of both nostrils at once, 15 times over the sink. Avoid the temptation to block off one nostril, or you could force water into the eustachian tubes, which run from the throat to the ears. Bend over the sink again to drain every drop of solution out of your deeper sinuses.

Repeat this nasal wash up to four times a day until your sinuses are clear. If you have a chronic problem, you can use it one to two times daily for several months.

"The solution will probably run down your throat or gag you until you get the hang of the treatment. I know it sounds horrible, but once you see the results, I'm quite sure you'll like it," says Dr. Bongiovanni.

—Bradley Bongiovanni, N.D., *is a naturopathic physician at Wellspace, a complementary health center in Cambridge, Massachusetts.*

STOCK UP ON OSCILLOCOCCINUM

Be sure to have a box of this famous remedy on hand at the first sign of the flu.

O scillococcinum is an obscure but sophisticated formula from the homeopathic medicine tradition. What makes it so unique is that it contains a number of different natural agents that target what your body needs to bring itself back into balance; then it can fight the flu at full force. Although it can make your symptoms more pronounced at first, it can actually speed up the healing process.

"It might be a new remedy for many Americans, but Oscillococcinum makes up nearly half of the European market for colds and flu (where homeopathic medicine in general is better known). "That's because it really is a very effective remedy," says Nancy Dunne Boggs, N.D.

Oscillococcinum comes in boxes containing three small tubes of tiny, sweet-tasting pellets. The dosage directions say to place an entire tube of pellets under your tongue every 6 hours. But it isn't necessary to take that much, Dr. Boggs explains. "As little as a scant ⅛ teaspoon is an effective dose."

For the best effect, it's very important to dose yourself within the first 12 to 48 hours of showing symptoms. Because of the imperative of timing, it's a good idea to have Oscillococcinum in your home rather than having to run out to buy it when you're getting sick.

—Nancy Dunne Boggs, N.D., *is a naturopathic physician practicing in Missoula, Montana, and founder of Bitterroot Natural Medicine, a botanical products company.*

CALL ON THE ALL-HERBAL FLU FIGHTER

Echinacea and the lesser-known medicinal herbs usnea, wild indigo, and elder are all tremendous flu fighters unto themselves. When used in combination, they can knock a virus out fast.

Over the past few years, echinacea has been making headline news for its promising ability to shorten the duration of colds and flu. Mary Bove, N.D., recommends using echinacea as the lead herb in an immune-boosting formula that helps your body defend itself in more ways than echinacea could do alone.

Wild indigo works in combination with echinacea to ease upper-respiratory tract infection. Usnea is a general immune stimulant that fights infection. Elder prevents the virus from reproducing, while also breaking up mucus and easing inflammation.

You'll probably buy each of these tinctures in 1-ounce bottles, available at health food stores or by mail order. Dr. Bove's formula calls for two parts echinacea to one part each of wild indigo, usnea, and elder. Use the entire 1-ounce bottle of echinacea, and half of each of the rest of the bottles. You now have your flu formula for the season.

Take a half teaspoon of the formula three times a day, Dr. Bove suggests. Start as soon as you suspect you're getting the flu. If you're not better after 3 weeks, discontinue the formula and call a doctor.

> **—Mary Bove, N.D.,** *is a naturopathic physician in Brattleboro, Vermont, and coauthor of* The Encyclopedia of Natural Healing for Children.

FIGHT FLU WITH GINGER AND GARLIC TEA

Whether your reason is temperance, or you're simply trying to avoid snoozing in the next morning, ginger and garlic are a good alternatives to over-the-counter cold and flu syrups.

For such a little root, ginger has heroic qualities. It certainly tastes a lot better than some of those alcohol-based syrups, and does far more than just suppress symptoms, says Tori Hudson, N.D.

Natural constituents in ginger are responsible for calming a cough, reducing pain and fever, and stopping inflammation. Ginger is a powerful tonic for nauseated stomachs. And without the help of alcohol, ginger also has a mild sedative effect—so you can rest.

Scientists have identified natural chemicals in ginger that have specific effects against fighting the most common family of cold viruses, the rhinovirus.

To double-whammy your sickness, bring on the bulb. Garlic is often recommended for the *prevention* of colds and flu, but it's not too late to take advantage of its germ-busting abilities once you start sneezing and coughing. "Garlic has potent antibiotic and antiviral properties that can keep a cold from hanging around," Dr. Hudson says.

Take this medicine in the form of warm tea.

Ginger and Garlic Tea

    1   piece (¾ inch) gingerroot, sliced
    2   cups water
    1   lemon wedge
    1   garlic clove
        Honey, to taste

In a pot, add the gingerroot slices to the water. Bring to a low boil, reduce the heat, and let simmer for 5 minutes. Strain the tea into a mug. Squeeze the lemon into the tea. Just before drinking, press in one clove of garlic. Add honey to sweeten the formula.

—Tori Hudson, N.D., *is a professor at the National College of Naturopathic Medicine and director of A Woman's Time naturopathic clinic in Portland, Oregon.*

Stopping the Spread

"Most cold and flu viruses are transmitted by touch."

—Peter Katona, M.D., *assistant professor of clinical medicine at the University of California, Los Angeles*

WASH YOUR HANDS OF COLDS AND FLU

This is the best infection stopper, hands-down. If you really want to decrease your chances of catching a cold or flu, start washing your hands—a lot.

Viruses can live from 1 to 3 hours on hands or infected objects, and colds in particular are most likely to be transmitted by touch. Hand-washing is the simplest and most effective way to avoid contracting a virus, because it sloughs off the skin particles that harbor viruses. Also, soap disrupts the cell walls of virus-laden cells, making it difficult for them to multiply, says infectious-disease expert Franklin R. Cockerill III, M.D.

A study presented to the American Academy of Family Physicians demonstrated the value of scrubbing up among a population of high-risk cold catchers: schoolchildren. When kids ages 5 to 12 were given four organized hand-washing breaks throughout the day, they had significantly fewer illnesses than those who didn't participate.

Adults can get just as much benefit from regular washing throughout the day, says Dr. Cockerill.

—Franklin R. Cockerill III, M.D., *is the chairperson of the division of clinical microbiology at the Mayo Clinic in Rochester, Minnesota.*

SEND THAT VIRUS
DOWN THE DRAIN

Know the art of scrubbing up. To stay
well during sniffle season, you need to be
a little more like a surgeon.

Here's how to improve your hand-washing, according to Franklin R. Cockerill III, M.D.

• The water should be at the hottest temperature you can tolerate, both when you rinse and when you initially wet your hands.

• Take your time to work up a good lather. Continue rubbing for 20 to 30 seconds. (Most people spend too little time at this—if you're one of them, try singing "Yankee Doodle" or another 30-second song to yourself while you're washing.)

• Skip the antibacterial soap; any plain soap will do. Antibacterial soaps have added chemicals such as triclosan, which are there to kill the germs that cause food-borne illnesses, but they probably aren't any more effective against viruses. What's more, continued overuse of these antibacterial chemicals might be adding to the growth of antibiotic-resistant bugs.

• Be sure to wash between your fingers and under your fingernails, the often-neglected nooks for bugs to hide. Use a small handbrush to facilitate getting under your nails.

• Rinse under running water until all the soap is gone.

• Dry thoroughly with a clean paper towel or an air dryer. The drying process itself will help get rid of extra germs.

There could be viruses on the faucet or door handle of a public restroom, but probably not enough to make a difference. If you're immune-compromised or the place is really filthy, use a paper towel to avoid direct contact.

—Franklin R. Cockerill III, M.D., *is the chairperson of the division of clinical microbiology at the Mayo Clinic in Rochester, Minnesota.*

JITTERBUG, DON'T SLOW DANCE

During the heart of cold and flu season, it's a good idea to maintain your personal space cushion to keep that bug at bay.

If a virus were colored chalk, the whole room at a party would be pigmented. There would be marks streaking up the furniture, glasses, and floor. But the darkest marks would be on the party-goers' hands, lips, and faces. If you actually *saw* them this way, you might be more cautious about getting too close.

"When you're touching something or someone infected with a virus, the germs are right there; they get on your hands and you touch your eyes or mouth, giving the infection a perfect passage into your bloodstream," says infectious disease specialist Peter Katona, M.D. Viruses do travel airborne, but far more cold and flu viruses are transmitted by touch rather than through coughs and sneezes. It's a more complicated process when a virus travels by air. The chances aren't as great that it would land in a vulnerable place and infect you, Dr. Katona adds.

When you kiss people or breathe in their faces, the virus can be transmitted directly. "Cold season just isn't the time to be greeting people with a hug and kiss. Even a simple handshake could make you sick, so be sure to wash your hands before touching them to your eyes, nose, or mouth," Dr. Katona says.

So there you have it—you finally have a reason to dodge Aunt Ethel from planting lipstick on your forehead this holiday season.

—Peter Katona, M.D., *is an assistant professor of clinical medicine at the University of California, Los Angeles.*

DON'T HANG YOURSELF OUT TO DRY

Heated, dry air irritates the throat and causes cracks in mucous membranes, which allows viruses an entry route. Protect yourself from Sahara-like air.

Dry air leaves you and your family open to infection. But there are several ways to make things moist.

"A room humidifier or a humidifying heater can really help, especially if someone in the house is already sick," says infectious disease specialist Peter Katona, M.D. If you have a wood stove, it's helpful to keep a big pot of water on top.

Dry air combined with frequent hand-washing can make already chapped skin on your hands all the more rough and cracked, another gateway to disease transmission. Use a moisturizer after washing your hands, says Dr. Katona. Just be careful not to re-infect your hands by touching a much-used dispenser without a tissue.

—Peter Katona, M.D., *is an assistant professor of clinical medicine at the University of California, Los Angeles.*

BLOW OFF YOUR COLD

Researchers discovered that inhaling a direct shot of hot air can shorten the course of the common cold and bring immediate relief to symptoms. You can administer your own hot air treatment by using a hair dryer.

If you've been exposed to someone with the sniffles, one preventive measure is to set a hair dryer on warm and simply breath the air through your nose. Directly heating your nasal mucosa just might kill a virus that's entering through the nose, says infectious disease specialist Peter Katona, M.D. Some viruses are more resistant to heat than others, but it's worth a try, he adds.

Backing up the hair dryer trick is a study done by the Medical Research Council Common Cold Unit at Harvard Hospital in England. Patients with acute nasal and upper-respiratory symptoms who breathed heated air from a test instrument for 20 minutes had roughly half the cold symptoms of volunteers who inhaled air closer to room temperature.

If 20 minutes seems like a long time to stand with a hair dryer in your face, some doctors say that even 2 or 3 minutes a night might help. But do it as long as you can, and as soon as you've been exposed to the virus.

The most important thing is not to let the air get too hot—that's not good for your mucous membranes. If it feels at all uncomfortable, put the dryer on a cooler setting or stop altogether.

—Peter Katona, M.D., *is an assistant professor of clinical medicine at the University of California, Los Angeles.*

REPLACE YOUR TOOTHBRUSH

When you have a cold or flu, replacing your toothbrush can help you win the germ war.

Toothbrushes are never something to be stingy about replacing. In fact, you should keep a few spare ones around for when you get sick. According to Richard T. Glass, D.D.S., Ph.D., viruses can last and produce disease on a toothbrush for 7 days.

Dr. Glass offers the following infection-avoiding recommendations.

• Replace your brush at the beginning, the most severe point, and the end of an illness.

• Dry toothbrushes harbor less bacteria than warm, wet ones. To help toothbrushes dry between use, store them uncovered, with the bristles up. Ideally, air them out in an area that's brighter and drier than the bathroom, such as your bedroom or kitchen window ledge.

- The sick person in the family should have his or her own tube of toothpaste, because germs can spread from the toothbrush to the tube.

If you're really worried about viruses on your brush, an ultraviolet device called the Purebrush will completely get rid of them, Dr. Glass says. It's available through Murdock Laboratories, 123 Primrose Road, Burlingame, CA 94010.

—Richard T. Glass, D.D.S., Ph.D., *is the director of the graduate program in forensic sciences at the Oklahoma State University College of Osteopathic Medicine in Tulsa.*

DON'T WAIT IN VAIN

What's the best way to pick up an illness? Go where all the sick people are.

Physicians' offices are sometimes the worst places to seek treatment for your cold or flu. It's not that your doctor isn't good at what he does; it's just that the waiting rooms are dens of infectious disease, says Sheldon Blau, M.D.

In fact, he contends, contracting a cold or flu could be the least of your worries, especially in a hospital waiting room. "Stay away from anybody coughing, sneezing, or vomiting, even if it means you don't get to take a seat," Dr. Blau recommends. "Try not to touch anything, and if you do, wash your hands well."

Because doctors' offices are often overwhelmed during flu season, call ahead to make sure appointments are running on time. It could save you precious minutes of avoiding a germy atmosphere.

Better yet, call your doctor before you head down to the office. For a common cold or flu without an overly high fever, your doctor can possibly advise you over the phone. Chances are, if you haven't developed a secondary infection, your doctor will confirm that all you need are some home remedies.

—**Sheldon Blau, M.D.,** *is a New York City physician and author of* How to Get Out of the Hospital Alive.

CONTAIN YOUR COUGH

When you have to cough in a crowded room, here's the best—and most polite—way to keep germs to yourself.

A cough usually occurs when excessive amounts of mucus build up and irritate your airways; its whole point is to rid you of infectious organisms. You need to get the stuff out, but at the same time you don't want to infect someone else with your illness.

When you feel a coughing spell coming on or you have a cough that you can't suppress, cough into your elbow so that you don't transmit the germs to your hands, says infectious disease specialist Peter Katona, M.D.

After you finish coughing, discipline yourself to wash your hands, especially if you do bring them to your face while coughing, he says. And if you have coughed on something else, wash it off.

—**Peter Katona, M.D.,** *is an assistant professor of clinical medicine at the University of California, Los Angeles.*

GO SOLO FOR SANITATION

Stay as far as possible from the madding crowds—especially if half the crowd is clinging to a facial tissue.

When you're running ragged and your resistance is down, it might not be the best time to be lingering in subway stations. There's a reason why subway passengers don't just *look* ill. "People commonly get sick in the wintertime because they're crowded together indoors," says infectious disease specialist Peter Katona, M.D.

Think about how a nasty flu bug (which is more easily transmitted through airborne particles than the cold virus) can travel from person to person in your office until everybody's had it at least once. Then there are day care centers, which seem to be disease incubators, he adds.

If you're coming down with something but have too much work to do to take any time off, Dr. Katona recommends that you work from home if at all possible. Really, you should allow yourself the extra rest needed to fight off illness. But even if you work at home, you avoid the added stress of a commute, not to mention the extra risk of being bombarded with other people's germs.

It might not be possible to avoid being in close quarters with virus carriers all the time, but one thing's for sure—if people are coughing or sneezing on you, it's time to go home.

—Peter Katona, M.D., *is an assistant professor of clinical medicine at the University of California, Los Angeles.*

BE PREPARED
WITH ASTRAGALUS

This herb is like having a personal top-notch coach who will whip your defenses into shape before the opposition has even formed—and keep you in your prime throughout the season.

Even before you break out your corduroy pants and retire garden tools to the shed, it's time to take this cold prevention herb. Call on the herb astragalus in the fall to avoid the woes of sniffle season. "Astragalus is a remarkable immune system strengthener. It helps the body produce and store more interferon within each cell. Interferon is a substance that tells disease-fighting white blood cells where the virus is attacking and how to stop it," says herbal expert Daniel Gagnon. Astragalus is considered such an effective immune strengthener that some doctors use it as part of cancer therapy.

"Since it has a pleasant taste, I prefer taking it as a tea infusion by using 1 teaspoon of the dried root per cup of boiling water and letting it steep for 10 to 15 minutes," he says. When you buy it in Asian markets and health food stores, it comes in bundles that look like tongue depressors. It can also be taken in capsule and tincture form by following label directions.

—Daniel Gagnon *is a founding member of the American Herbalists Guild, executive director of the Botanical Research and Education Institute, and owner of Herbs, Etc., in Santa Fe, New Mexico.*

TRASH YOUR TISSUES

Clean up now and lower your risk of re-infection later. Besides, it's rude to expose the rest of the house to crumpled, germy tissues.

True, it can get boring lying in bed all day with the sniffles, but don't occupy yourself by trying to slam-dunk your used Kleenex into the wastebasket across the room—that is, unless you're a perfect shot.

Caretakers who have to retrieve your foul shots are in jeopardy of coming down with your bug (not to mention that they might become disgusted with you and not bring you any more chicken soup).

Resist the temptation to scatter your germs playing Magic Johnson, and do a harmless crossword puzzle instead. Seriously, a sick person's used tissues should be treated like the infectious waste that it is, says infectious disease specialist Peter Katona, M.D. Throw tissues out maturely, into a garbage pail lined with a trash bag, and dispose of the trash bags frequently.

It's also no good to stick them into your pockets where someone else is going to have to retrieve them to do the laundry. Don't leave them on the nightstand or pillow either, where the virus can live for several hours.

"It's often very simple things that make the difference in whether or not someone gets sick," adds Dr. Katona.

—Peter Katona, M.D., *is an assistant professor of clinical medicine at the University of California, Los Angeles.*

Alternative Options

Healers Who Can Help

A true advantage to using home remedies is that you can take healing into your own hands. But sometimes you need extra help.

Maybe your immunity is so low that you seem to develop a cold when someone in the other room sneezes. Or maybe you're one of those people who are still in bed with the flu when the rest of the family has bounced back—yet you had it first.

The alternative medicine approach is to build your natural defenses rather than treat your symptoms. So if you seem to develop more colds than a day care teacher at the North Pole, you might benefit from a series of visits with an alternative practitioner who can develop a long-term strategy for better overall health.

Alternative experts are known for inquiring about your lifestyle, relationships, and diet in order to get to the root of low immunity. While your family doctor doesn't have much to give you for avoiding the next cold, your alternative practitioner might offer nutrition, herbs, bodywork, and stress-reduction techniques as support. She might also want to team up with other alternative practitioners, such as those in her practice or holistic medical association, to offer you the most well-rounded treatment.

You might also want to visit an alternative practitioner if your cold or flu won't go away. By using natural remedies, such as those recommended in this book, your cold or flu should improve significantly in a week or less. If you aren't getting better, have your family doctor or holistic physician rule out a more serious illness. If you don't have secondary infections or a major illness, call on alternative healers.

Many alternative healers have the training to design powerful natural medicine formulas that address your specific symptoms. They might provide a special combination of herbal teas, an essential oil mixture, or homeopathic pills to take at specific times of the day. And the skilled hands of an acupuncturist or massage therapist can also give you the relief you simply can't find in a drugstore.

Unfortunately, just because a person calls himself an "alternative medicine practitioner" or maybe a "holistic healer" does not make him credible. Use this guide not only to help you choose a modality for your cold and flu problems but also to help you locate a healer who is qualified—so you can get the kind of result *and care* that you might be seeking.

Acupressure

Although acupressure can't *cure* a cold, it's a therapy that can help you get better quicker, relieve pain, and increase your resistance to future colds, says acupressure expert Michael Reed Gach, Ph.D.

Many variations have developed over the years, but all acupressure is based on the same basic principle. Finger or hand pressure is used to stimulate points on the body that activate what Chinese medical practitioners call Qi—the body's living energy—which can restore balance to an unhealthy body.

You'll find that an acupressurist will stimulate points near the area of trouble (local points) with points that seem to have no obvious connection to the immediate problem (trigger points), says Dr. Gach. One "local point" for treating a cough is between the shoulder blade and the spine, an area that often spasms during a coughing fit. But then there are trigger points farther away from the area of trouble that work because energetic meridian pathways connect the points, he explains. One surprising "trigger point" to relieve congestion is on the elbow crease outside of your forearm.

From a book or class, you can learn some basic pressure points yourself, such as squeezing the mound between your thumb and forefinger to relieve a sinus headache. But trained acupressurists know hundreds of pressure points that constitute a highly sophisticated healing sequence—not to mention some points you simply can't reach yourself!

Practitioners who might offer acupressure treatment include Shiatsu and other massage therapists, licensed acupuncturists, doctors of oriental medicine (O.M.D.'s), family doctors, and naturopaths. In some states the practitioner must be certified or licensed to practice. Membership in the American Oriental Bodywork Therapy Association is a good assurance of competency.

For more information on how to locate a qualified acupressure practitioner, contact the American Oriental Bodywork Therapy Association, 6801 Jerico Turnpike, Syosset, NY 11791.

Acupuncture

Prepare to be prodded when you visit an acupuncturist, who will run his or her hands along your body, feeling for tender spots. Like acupressurists, acupuncturists believe this tenderness is caused by obstructions in the energetic meridians of your body that hinder the flow of Qi. In order to enhance the body's innate healing abilities, acupuncturists use hair-thin needles to stimulate precise points along this ancient map of energetic pathways.

Acupuncturists might stimulate certain points to clear phlegm from the nose and lungs, for example, or insert needles to remedy all-over malaise during a flu outbreak.

The World Health Organization recognizes acupuncture as a treatment for the following cold and flu-related problems: sore throats, sinusitis, chest infections, and headaches. Practitioners say that their healing system is an excellent method for cutting short all major symptoms of colds and flu.

The actual protocol—how many needles are used, how deeply they are inserted, and how long they are left in—depends on the diagnosis and the preference of the practitioner. So do the frequency and duration of treatments. The needles might sting slightly upon insertion, but the pain quickly goes away. Because they are so fine, there is seldom any bleeding, except in an area with a lot of blood vessels like the hands.

State laws vary on who can practice acupuncture, but it is estimated that approximately 15,000 acupuncturists are licensed nationwide. The most common practitioners are doctors of oriental medicine (O.M.D.'s) and general licensed acupuncturists (L.Ac.'s), but many M.D.'s and D.O.'s are also trained.

Look for the following qualification in a practitioner: certification by the National Certification Commission for Acupuncture and Oriental Medicine (NCCAOM). In order to become certified, these practitioners must finish an intensive training program and pass a certifying exam in the states in which they practice.

For a directory of practitioners, contact the American Academy of Medical Acupuncture (AAMA), 5820 Wilshire Boulevard, Suite 500, Los Angeles, CA 90036.

Aromatherapy

As simple as it might seem to plug in a potpourri pot or drop some floral-scented liquid into your bath, trained aromatherapists say there is a real skill to using distilled plant essences called essential oils. By consulting with an expert, you should receive the maximum effect from what essential oils have to offer—in two words, deep comfort. Aromatherapists can help you get relief from coughs, congestion, irritability, aches, pains, and the general malaise that accompanies colds and flu.

Among the skills that the healers can offer is recommending which oils, among the hundreds of options, have the right properties to bring you relief from your specific symptoms. Aromatherapists will also discuss with you the amount of oil necessary to achieve your desired effect, the length of time to use it, safety precautions, how to select premium ingredients, and what method of administration to use. (Oils are commonly administered through inhalation in steamy water, sprayed into the air, massaged into the skin, diluted in a bath, or dropped into hot and cold compresses.)

On a more advanced level than simply making you *feel* better, aromatherapists claim that they have remedies to boost your immune system, which helps *prevent* colds and flu, as well as formulas to actually *treat* your virus by way of its antimicrobial properties.

Medical studies proving this modality's effectiveness are scarce. But aromatherapists consider their work a science—combining botany, chemistry, biology, and psychology. Practitioners explain, for instance, that certain essential oils ease pain and inflammation because their chemicals stimulate the adrenal glands, which produce steroid-like hormones. The bottom line is that the greater depth of understanding the aromatherapist has regarding the use of oils, the more possibilities open up as to the relief and healing she can bring you.

Unfortunately, there's no formal licensing procedure for aromatherapists in the United States, but you will find that it's offered by alternative practitioners with licences in fields including chiropractic, psychology, and massage therapy, as well as by herbalists and people who simply specialize in aromatherapy.

For more information, contact the National Association for Holistic Aromatherapy, P.O. Box 17622, Boulder, CO 80308.

Herbal Medicine

Herbal remedies might be the ideal treatment for colds and flu. There are hundreds of readily available plants that can address every stage of a cold or flu symptom. In addition, they present virtually no side effects, compared to the grogginess, nervousness, or dependency that can result from over-the-counter medication, says Daniel Gagnon, a founding member of the American Herbalists Guild.

But because of the popularity of herbal medicine, it's easy to become overwhelmed by the array of teas, capsules, and tinctures on the market, as well as by the glut of herbal advice in the media. Based on your symptoms, a professional herbalist can help you make the best selection of herbs or herbal combinations, and will know when in the cold or flu cycle to take which herb.

An herbalist prescribes a *preventive* herb early in the cold and flu season to protect you from getting the bug altogether. If you do get sick, at the first sign of symptoms she selects herbs, such as famous echinacea and elderberry remedies, to provide a *first line of defense*. These herbs often can stop the virus before it fully develops. If you don't see an herbalist until you already have a full-blown virus, she has an array of plants that work as *symptom relievers*, from reducing inflammation of the mucous membrane to breaking up lung congestion. Even for secondary infections that develop out of a cold or flu, such as sinusitis or ear infection, herbalists have an arsenal of remedies that can serve as *natural antibiotics*.

As consumer interest in herbal medicine has grown in the United States, so does the ease of finding a practitioner. Some M.D.'s are incorporating herbalists into their practices. Other M.D.'s themselves are being schooled in herbal healing at medical institutions such as Harvard, Columbia, and the University of California.

In total, there are approximately 15,000 to 20,000 health care professionals in this country who prescribe medicinal herbs—including general herbalists, family doctors, naturopathic doctors, and doctors of oriental medicine.

To locate a qualified herbalist in your area, contact the American Herbalists Guild, P.O. Box 70, Roosevelt, UT 84066.

Homeopathy

Hippocrates, the founding father of modern medicine, espoused that an individual prescription should be developed for each individual patient. Homeopathy exquisitely follows Hippocrates's principle. According to homeopaths, it's essential to recognize that each person experiences a cold or flu in his or her unique way.

For example, the person with the early stages of a cold—characterized by slow onset, aching, loss of appetite, chills, and a desire to be left alone—will need an entirely different remedy than a person whose cold came on quicker and who has intense sneezing, a runny nose that burns the upper lip, and a desire to be comforted.

To evaluate you, doctors take into account details such as the time of day when your pain is worse or better, the current weather, what foods you crave, if you have chills or sweats, and even what emotions you are feeling. From there, they might choose from hundreds of remedies, according to a system that has been shown to work since the late eighteenth century. An array of hospitals and medical schools have been based on the homeopathic system, developed by the German medical pioneer, Samuel Hahnemann, M.D.

Using such precise medicine, homeopaths can ideally direct such deep and efficient healing of your cold or flu that it might also prevent you from getting another virus anytime soon. And when prescribed correctly, by a trained homeopath, homeopathy can heal you quickly, without side effects, such as drowsiness or irritability associated with prescription or over-the-counter medications. This is because the medicines are such extreme dilutions of mineral, plant, and animal ingredients that they don't disrupt your system.

Even if you have never heard of a homeopath before, there might be more of them than you think. Approximately 3,000 homeopaths practice nationwide—1,000 of them are medical doctors or osteopaths. The rest include naturopaths, nurse-practitioners, dentists, licensed acupuncturists, and chiropractors.

Check to see whether your practitioner has completed in-depth training, which includes 500 or more hours in homeopathic philosophy, methodology, and clinical training, which are offered by various educational organizations across the country. Those who train extensively earn some of the following initials in their title: DHt, DI.Hom., N.D., DHANP, or CCH.

For more information, contact the National Center for Homeopathy, 801 N. Fairfax Street #306, Alexandria, VA 22314.

Naturopathic Medicine

Many people who see naturopathic physicians say it is because they like the variety of options they are offered. Doctors of naturopathy mix and match customized, nondrug treatments. So for your cold and flu symptoms, a naturopath might focus on gentle dietary and lifestyle adjustments such as juice therapy, boosting your vitamin intake, relaxation techniques, and heating compresses to the throat, in addition to taking herbal or homeopathic medicine.

Naturopathic doctors who are accepted into the American Association of Naturopathic Physicians (AANP) have attended a medical school where they spent as much time studying the basic sciences—anatomy, physiology, biochemistry, neurology, pathology, and diagnostic techniques—as their colleagues in conventional medical school. In addition, they take courses in homeopathy, therapeutic nutrition, hydrotherapy, botanical medicine, spinal manipulation, and other alternative therapeutic modalities that are not required for medical doctor degrees.

Seek out a member of the AANP to be sure a naturopath has had the proper in-depth training. For a directory of members, contact the American Association of Naturopathic Physicians (AANP), 601 Valley Street, Suite 105, Seattle, WA 98109.

For more information on these and other alternative healing modalities, contact the Office of Alternative Medicine (OAM) at the National Institutes of Health (NIH). Write for their "General Information Package" at OAM Clearinghouse, P.O. Box 8218, Silver Spring, MD 20907.

Index